# Vaccines after Cancer

## TAKING CONTROL

BC PUBLISHING
SYDNEY, AUSTRALIA

**Your vaccination guide through cancer treatment and beyond**

TAKING

Second Edition

# Vaccines after Cancer

# TAKING CONTROL

Professor John Boyages, MD, PhD

BC PUBLISHING

SYDNEY, AUSTRALIA

*Vaccines after Cancer: Taking Control*

BC Publishing
PO Box 568 Beecroft, NSW 2119, Australia
www.bcpublish.com
bcpublishers@gmail.com



Published in Australia. Written in UK English.
1st edition (2021)
2nd edition (2025)

ISBN (Print): 978-1-7640718-2-6 (KDP Standard)
978-1-7640718-3-3 (KDP Premium)

ISBN (ebook): 978-1-7640718-8-8



Important: The contents of this book should not be used in place of a visit, call, or consultation with and advice given by your physician or other healthcare providers. Talk to your doctor or pharmacist before taking any prescription or over-the-counter drugs (including herbal medicines or supplements). You should never disregard professional medical advice or delay seeking it because of something you read in this book or on any website. While every effort has been made to ensure that the material in this book is accurate at the time of publication, discoveries are often made, and treatment practices may ultimately change, update, or invalidate some of the information presented here. Any use of this book is at the reader's discretion. While every effort has been made to ensure the information is accurate, complete, and current, BC Publishing and the author do not guarantee and assume no legal liability or responsibility for the accuracy, currency, or completeness of the information.

Reference to external resources in this publication should not be taken as an endorsement or recommendation of any third-party products or services offered, and the views or recommendations provided by these external resources do not necessarily reflect those of BC Publishing. Note that a healthcare professional should always be consulted regarding your specific situation.

Subjects: Cancer; Vaccination; COVID-19; Influenza; Shingles; Patient education; Survivorship

# DEDICATION

To my nephew Dr Costa Boyages, who strongly suggested I get vaccinated to protect against pneumonia, shingles and whooping cough after my cancer treatment, and who inspired me to write this book.

# Praise for *Vaccines after Cancer: Taking Control*

John Boyages has written a must-read book for patients with cancer wanting the latest advice about vaccinations before and after treatment. His book is easy to read, yet contains well-researched information about COVID-19, influenza, shingles, and other vaccines. This is an excellent resource not only for patients and their families, but also for general practitioners, nurses, and oncologists.

**Professor Peter Collignon AM,** Infectious Diseases Physician and Microbiologist, Canberra Hospital and Australian National University

Completing anti-cancer therapy is not the end, but rather a beginning. It marks the commencement of life as a cancer survivor, which is a privileged and fantastic position, but a situation whereby medical care is often more complex. Although preventative medical care post-cancer therapy is important, it is often not given the importance that it deserves. John Boyages has addressed this breach by writing a comprehensive and practical guide to vaccination post-cancer therapy. Vaccination is amongst the most effective tools in modern medicine, and it is vitally important that this aspect of preventative medical care is not overlooked in cancer survivors. I commend this guide to cancer survivors, carers, and health professionals alike.

**Dr Ian Irving,** Clinical Haematologist and Group Medical Director, Icon Cancer Centre

In line with his other excellent books, John has done it again. This is an insightful, timely, well-referenced, excellent review of the current vaccine-related issues facing our patients today. It is a clear, easy-to-read, practical guide to empowering patients and their carers to make appropriate, safe, and evidence-based decisions. Well done. Thank you!

**Professor Gavin Marx,** Medical Oncologist, Northern Haematology Oncology Group; Director, Clinical Trials Unit, Sydney Adventist Hospital; Clinical Director, San Integrated Cancer Centre

As a patient of John Boyages, I was so grateful for his professionalism and for the compassion and clarity with which he explained the options available to me during my breast cancer treatment. All these qualities are evident in this wonderfully practical book. John has the unique ability to convey complex medical information in a manner that makes it both digestible and easy to apply for the layperson.

**Liane Moriarty,** Australian author

# Contents

# About the author

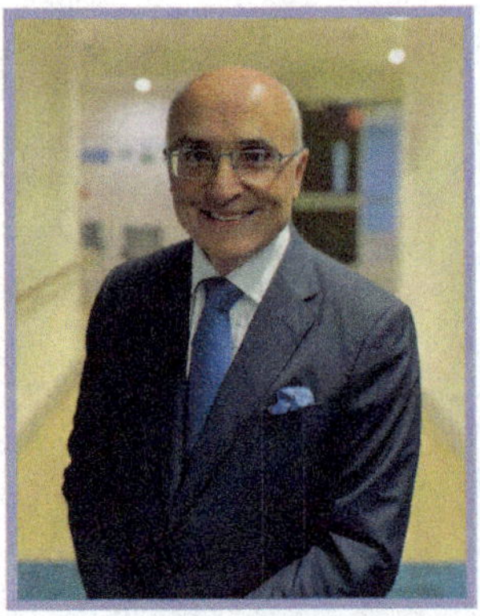

Professor John Boyages, MD, PhD is a cancer specialist with 40 years of experience in breast cancer management. He is a radiation oncologist at Icon Cancer Centre, and founding director and honorary professor of the Australian Lymphoedema Education, Research and Treatment (ALERT) Centre.

Following his fellowship at Harvard Medical School, John was appointed as a specialist radiation oncologist at Westmead Hospital in 1989, and in 1993 he founded Australia's largest free breast screening program in Sydney's west. In 1995, he established and directed the Westmead Breast Cancer Institute, a comprehensive breast cancer program. John established the ALERT lymphoedema program at Macquarie University in 2012.

John has published more than 200 research and clinical articles and is a reviewer for multiple international journals. In 2010, John published his bestselling and award-winning book, *Breast Cancer: Taking Control*, for patients with breast cancer. In 2014, he published *DCIS of the Breast: Taking Control,* followed by *Male Breast Cancer: Taking Control* in 2015. In 2021, he continued the series with *Vaccines after Cancer: Taking Control* and in 2025 published *Lymphoedema: Taking Control.*

In addition to his research, John works as a radiation oncologist providing expert care to patients with breast cancer in Sydney. He enjoys spending spare moments with his family and friends, enjoys bushwalking and is learning bridge and oil painting.

In 2017, John was appointed a Member in the General Division of the Order of Australia (AM) for his significant service to medicine.

## ACKNOWLEDGEMENTS

I would especially like to thank my wife, Dianne, for her ongoing patience and support. Thanks also to my beautiful children, Fiona and Peter, my son-in-law David and daughter-in-law Lauren, for their ongoing humour, support and understanding. Special mention also to my beautiful grandchildren: Jack, Anna, Lily, Elsie, Samuel and Florence.

Expert medical review of the first edition was undertaken by Professor Peter Collignon AM, infectious diseases physician and microbiologist at the Canberra Hospital and professor at the Australian National University.

Thank you also to Dr Csilla Hasovits and Dr Josie Rutovitz from the Northern Haematology Oncology Group; Dr Costa Boyages, general practitioner in Nowra and Bomaderry, and Dr Ian Irving, clinical haematologist at the ICON Cancer Centre, for their expert peer review.

I am also grateful to my long-standing patient Sue Hume for her thorough review of the first edition. All reviews greatly improved the book.

# Introduction

The day I was awarded an Order of Australia in 2017 was a bittersweet moment for me, as it came one day after I received my first dose of chemotherapy. My treatment for Hodgkin's lymphoma involved an intensive course of chemotherapy and radiation therapy, with multiple hospital admissions and complications. Finally, after eight months off work, I too became a 'cancer survivor'.

My treatment team didn't talk to me about vaccination, and I suspect many of you are in the same situation. In late 2020, my nephew Dr Costa Boyages, a general practitioner, called me and said I needed to be vaccinated for shingles, pneumonia, and whooping cough, especially because of my previous cancer treatment. To make matters worse, we were in the middle of the **COVID-19 pandemic**, and many of my patients – recently treated for cancer – started contacting me, anxious about whether it was safe to have the AstraZeneca vaccine due to reports of a rare blood-clotting condition.

As a cancer survivor, you may be more prone to catching an infection, and you may produce an inadequate response due to your possibly weakened **immune system**. The time for your immunity to recover after treatment varies and will be longer if you have had intensive chemotherapy or a bone marrow transplant.

A very common question patients have asked me is, "Can I have the flu shot?" In 2020 that question was replaced by "Should I have the COVID-19 shot?" and "Can the COVID-19 **vaccine** cause clots given I'm taking hormonal treatment for my breast cancer?" There are also many other questions patients ask about timing vaccinations around their cancer treatments.

This book aims to help you or your family member understand:

- which vaccines to have before or after your cancer treatment
- the difference between live and inactivated vaccines and the ones to avoid
- how to reduce your chances of an unwanted infection
- what complications to look out for after vaccination
- how to avoid lymphoedema after a vaccine
- all about COVID-19 vaccines in the context of a previous cancer diagnosis
- how to avoid infections such as shingles, pneumonia, and whooping cough.

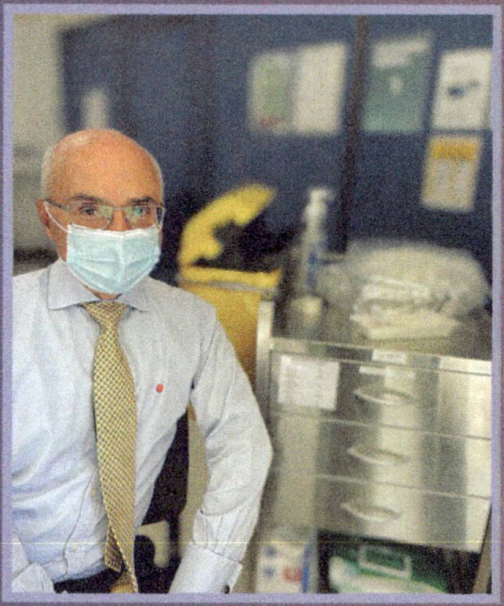

John having his first dose of the AstraZeneca COVID-19 vaccine in March 2021.

The book includes real-life patient stories, key web links, figures and tables underpinned by an extensive reference list.

Glossary terms are in bold when used in the text for the first time.

# 1

# UNDERSTANDING VACCINES

## WHAT IS A VACCINE?

A vaccine is given by injection under your skin or into your muscle to build up your body's immune system to fight a future, unencountered, harmful disease. The body's immune system protects us every day by identifying specific molecules called **antigens** in harmful bugs and producing fighting proteins called **antibodies**.

Special white blood cells called **lymphocytes** also target antigens for destruction. Some lymphocytes known as **T cells** retain memory and can generate long-lasting immunity. Some vaccines require more than one dose, called a **booster**, given weeks or months apart.

Some vaccines use a live but weakened **virus** to ensure the body produces immunity against the offending bug. This approach allows you to develop antibodies to attack the actual virus or bug if you are unlucky enough to be infected. Other vaccines are inactivated rather than live, and these are generally safe for patients with cancer. Vaccines may be **monovalent** or **polyvalent**. A monovalent vaccine contains a single strain of a single antigen (e.g., measles vaccine), whereas a polyvalent vaccine contains two or more strains of the same antigen (e.g., some flu and pneumonia vaccines).

Some vaccines are combined, which means that different antigens are combined into a single injection (e.g., dTpa combines tetanus, diphtheria, and pertussis antigens). **Combined vaccines** can be helpful to overcome logistic constraints or a person's fear of having multiple injections.

Some **bacteria** are protected by a polysaccharide (sugar) capsule when infecting humans. This capsule helps the organism evade the human defence systems, especially in infants and young children. **Polysaccharide vaccines** create a response against the molecules on the bacteria's capsule. These molecules are small and often do not produce a robust immune response and tend to induce only short-term immunity.

## WHAT MAKES AN IDEAL VACCINE?

The World Health Organization (WHO) noted that vaccine manufacturers strive to develop vaccines that:

- are effective in preventing or reducing the severity of infectious disease
- provide long-term protection against the disease
- achieve immunity with as few doses as possible

- provide the maximum number of antigens that confer the broadest protection against infection
- cause no side-effects, or mild side-effects only
- are stable and long-lasting at temperature extremes
- are available through mass production
- are affordable for at-risk populations.

## WHAT IS A 'LIVE' VACCINE?

A few vaccines contain a weakened version of live viruses. They are sometimes called live **attenuated vaccines**. Attenuation means taking an infectious agent and altering it to make it harmless or less infectious. The idea is that if a vaccinated person is exposed to the actual virus, it will cause no disease, or only a very mild form of it.

The advantage of a **live vaccine** is that it generates a strong **immune response**. The disadvantage is that it can cause potentially life-threatening infections in people with weak immune systems. If your immunity is low, be sure to talk to your doctor before anyone in your family (such as your children or other household members) gets any live vaccines.

Some examples of live vaccines include:

- MMR vaccine for measles, mumps, and rubella
- BCG (bacille Calmette–Guérin) vaccine for tuberculosis
- Yellow fever vaccine
- Oral typhoid vaccine
- Intranasal influenza vaccine (e.g., Fluenz Tetra/FluMist® nasal spray)
- Imojev® vaccine for Japanese encephalitis.

You won't need most of these vaccines unless you're travelling to an at-risk country or region. Avoid them for at least six months after completing your cancer treatment.

## WHAT IS AN 'INACTIVATED' VACCINE?

**Inactivated vaccines** are made from viruses or bacteria killed through a physical (e.g., heat or radiation) or chemical process. You can safely have an inactivated vaccine if you have had cancer. These vaccines may not work as well if you have a weakened immune system.

Inactivated vaccines usually include those for:

- COVID-19
- Diphtheria, tetanus, pertussis +/- polio (combined)
- Influenza/flu (when given by injection)
- Rabies
- Cholera
- Typhoid (when given by injection)
- Meningococcus
- Tick-borne encephalitis
- Japanese encephalitis (JEspect®)
- Hepatitis A and B (available separately or combined)
- Pneumococcal disease
- Meningococcal disease
- Respiratory syncytial virus (RSV)
- Shingles.

## WHAT IS HERD IMMUNITY?

Not everyone can (or wants to) be vaccinated. These people can still be protected if they live in and around people who are vaccinated. When many people in the community are vaccinated, the virus or bug has a hard time circulating from person to person, as the vaccine protects most people. However, no vaccine provides 100% protection, and herd immunity does not work for everyone who is not vaccinated.

Herd immunity can also occur when many people in the population have recovered from a disease and have developed antibodies against future infection. For example, in a study of 32 survivors of the 1918 influenza pandemic aged 91 to 101 years (aged 2–12 in 1918), the participants still had signs of reactivity to the virus strain, showing that their immune system was on standby for a potential second outbreak (Yu, 2008).

**For more on herd immunity, see https://www.mayoclinic.org/diseases-conditions/coronavirus/in-depth/herd-immunity-and-coronavirus/art-20486808.**

Before the COVID-19 vaccine was discovered, we saw the disastrous consequences of relying on herd immunity in Sweden, where the infection rate from the disease and the subsequent number of deaths was higher than in other Scandinavian countries. What is still unclear is whether a previous COVID-19 infection gives you sustainable immunity. More research is needed to determine the protective effect of antibodies on the virus for those infected.

## WHAT ARE COMMON SIDE-EFFECTS AFTER VACCINATION?

Side-effects after vaccination are generally classified as local (meaning the reaction is at the vaccination site or nearby lymph node areas) or systemic (meaning that the reaction takes the form of generalised body symptoms).

## LOCAL REACTIONS

Most vaccines are given under the skin (**intradermal**) or into a large muscle (**intramuscular**) such as your upper arm. Some vaccines cause local swelling and pain at the injection site. These reactions can occur within a few hours of your vaccination and typically resolve within two to seven days. Moving your shoulder (deltoid) muscle after vaccination into your upper arm immediately after and for several hours after your vaccination may reduce pain. If your arm is sore, an ice pack can help reduce pain and swelling. Others find that a heat pack relaxes the muscle. See what works best for you.

The condition of swollen, tender lymph nodes is generally called **lymphadenitis**. Feeling a lump under your arm can be frightening. If the swelling is tender and has turned up within two to four weeks after your vaccination, it is most likely due to your body fighting the vaccine and creating antibodies. If you have a mammogram or a PET-CT scan, the lymph gland may be visible and falsely alarm the radiologist. Ask your doctor to specify which arm you had your recent vaccination in on any relevant imaging referral form and notify the imaging technician.

If the lump becomes redder and more painful, it may be a sign of infection, but this is extremely rare after a vaccination. See your surgeon or family doctor for a trial of antibiotics. If the lump is also getting larger, see your doctor, who may order an ultrasound and perhaps a fine needle or core biopsy. I would observe the swelling for a few weeks and take some paracetamol/acetaminophen (Panadol/Tylenol) if you have pain. Avoid aspirin and anti-inflammatory drugs.

There have been a few rare case reports of arm **lymphoedema** becoming worse in patients who developed a nasty skin and tissue reaction to a

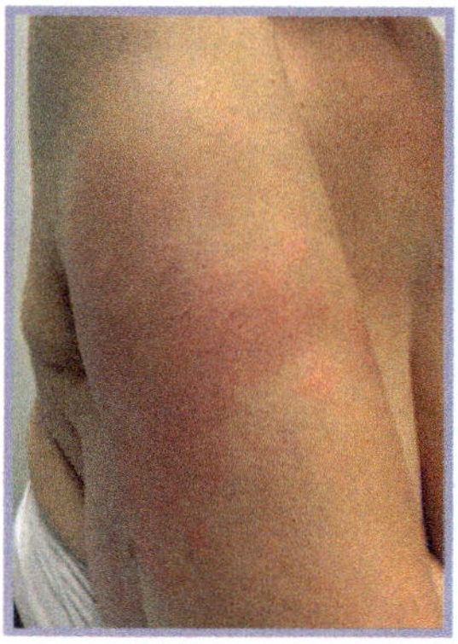

**Figure 1.1**

Redness and probable infection occurring two weeks after COVID-19 vaccination on the same side as breast cancer treatment six years earlier.

vaccine, so it's best to have the vaccine in your unaffected arm (Lee, 2012). If you have had treatment on both your breasts, you should have the vaccine in your thigh or buttocks.

In 2020, one of my patients, whom I had treated for right-sided breast cancer about six years earlier, returned for her annual check-up. She mentioned that her right upper arm became sore two weeks after her COVID-19 vaccination **(Figure 1.1)**. Although she had only received radiation to the right breast without surgery to the lymph nodes in her armpit, she seemed to have developed some mild swelling in her lower arm. I started her on antibiotics and referred her to our lymphoedema team.

## GENERALISED REACTIONS

Generalised or systemic reactions are also usually minor. These include headache, fatigue, muscle aches and pains, a mild fever and, in rare cases, loss of appetite.

Severe reactions are rarely life-threatening and are highly uncommon. If they occur, they are often due to an allergy to a specific component in the vaccine such as preservatives, stabilisers or ingredients called adjuvants which help amplify the immune response.

Early signs of **anaphylaxis** (a severe allergic reaction) include widespread, generalised redness or itching of the skin, swelling (hives), breathing difficulties and a sense of distress. Most vaccine centres or doctors will keep you under observation for at least 15 minutes after your vaccination so that they can watch out for these symptoms. On rare occasions, they will give adrenaline for a severe allergic reaction. If you are prone to allergies, consider going to a larger venue such as a hospital-based vaccination centre or a larger medical clinic with more doctors and nurses around.

Severe allergic reactions can occur a few hours after vaccination, so call your local emergency number for urgent assistance if you have any of these symptoms. It's not a bad idea to stay close to somebody at work or home and let them know you have been vaccinated.

# 2

# PROTECTING YOURSELF AFTER CANCER

## HOW DO I REDUCE MY CHANCE OF GETTING AN INFECTION?

Following cancer treatment, it is crucial to get back to your everyday life. One thing we have learned from the COVID-19 pandemic is that social isolation reduces the risk of infection. Before the pandemic, my mother had been admitted to hospital most years with a bad cold or flu that often required oxygen. However, in 2020 during the lockdown in Australia, we kept her protected at home, and she remained well. In Australia, the incidence of influenza-like illnesses was extremely low in 2020 and the first half of 2021. We continued to shop online for my mother after the pandemic as a way to restrict her movements a little more, particularly during the colder months.

The following advice can help to reduce your risk of infection, and many of these suggestions also apply if you have just finished your chemotherapy. If you have just had surgery, or radiation with or without hormonal treatment, your chances of infection are usually no more than the average population.

- Avoid busy indoor places, including crowded public transport, and wear a mask, particularly in winter.
- Wear a face mask if you cannot maintain social distance in crowded indoor spaces.
- Wash your hands before and after close contact with people and animals.
- When washing your hands is difficult, use a hand sanitiser with at least 60% alcohol content.
- Wear gloves to prevent skin cuts and reduce the risk of infection, e.g., in the garden.
- Wear shoes outdoors.
- Wear a cap when swimming in unsafe water to protect your ears and prevent infection. Appropriate earplugs will also protect your ear canals. Use a hairdryer to dry your external ear canal rather than cotton buds, which can irritate the skin and encourage an infection (Sander, 2001).
- If drinking water may not be safe, drink bottled water and don't use ice (e.g., when travelling overseas).

- Don't touch animal faeces or fluids, which can transmit disease. **Toxoplasmosis** can be transmitted from cat faeces and some undercooked meats. Although it may not cause any symptoms, minor symptoms such as fever, a sore throat, swollen lymph nodes, or generalised aches can occur. Toxoplasmosis can be dangerous if your immunity is low during or just after chemotherapy.

Now, I don't want you thinking that you will constantly be at risk of infection after treatment, and I don't like to suggest you should wrap yourself in cotton wool. However, these suggestions are common sense, particularly if your immunity has been affected by chemotherapy.

**For more information on preventing toxoplasmosis, see https://www.cdc.gov/toxoplasmosis/prevention**

## IS MY IMMUNITY REDUCED AFTER CANCER TREATMENT?

After cancer treatment, many people have some reduction in immunity. How much – and for how long – will depend on your cancer type, treatment intensity, and other illnesses or medications. Treatments such as recent chemotherapy, radiation to areas with a lot of bone marrow, high-dose steroids, and stem-cell/CAR T-cell therapy can temporarily lower the amount of lymphocytes (B and T cells) in your body, which are key for fighting infection and forming vaccine protection. That's why some vaccines are timed around treatment, and why your treatment team may recommend revaccination once your immune system recovers.

A cancer patient is considered highly **immunocompromised** if they have:

- metastatic cancer (cancer that has spread)
- a **haematological malignancy** (blood cancer)
- received chemotherapy or radiation therapy in the past three months
- received the equivalent of ≥ 20 mg prednisone daily for two or more weeks
- received a bone marrow transplant in the past two years, or more than two years ago if there is ongoing evidence of **graft-versus-host disease (GVHD)**.

The U.S. Centers for Disease Control and Prevention (CDC) offers advice for clinicians on vaccinating people with 'altered immunocompetence', including cancer patients receiving immunosuppressive treatment like chemotherapy or radiation. The CDC suggests giving vaccines before **immunosuppression** where possible; inactivated vaccines can be given during or after treatment, though responses may be lower. If a live vaccine is needed, wait at least three to six months after cancer treatment, or up to a year for certain medications (lymphocyte-depleting agents). Short courses of immunosuppressive steroids generally require at least a month before giving a live vaccine (CDC, 2024a). The timing will vary depending on your individual circumstances, so check with your oncologist or an **immunisation** specialist.

If you are able to get vaccinated before your treatment, the recommended timing is at least four weeks before immunosuppression for live vaccines, and at least two weeks for inactivated vaccines (CDC, 2025a).

**See https://www.cdc.gov/yellow-book/hcp/travelers-with-additional-considerations/immunocompromised-travelers.html for more information.**

There are two concerns for cancer patients. Firstly, a live vaccine may make you very sick, and in rare cases, it could cause death if your immunity is very depressed. Secondly, if your immune system is depressed, it may not be able to mount an adequate response to the vaccine, leaving you unprotected.

Immunity is unlikely to be affected for patients who have localised radiation to the breast (without treating the surrounding lymph nodes). For radiation fields that treat large reserves of bone marrow (such as the pelvis or the spine), it is best to wait at least three months before you have any new vaccines, but check with your oncologist first.

If you are on long-term, low-dose corticosteroid therapy on its own or combined with other immunosuppressive therapy, consider delaying vaccination and consulting with both your treating doctor and an immunisation specialist when considering live vaccines.

## WHAT DO I DO ABOUT VACCINATION IF I HAVE LYMPHOEDEMA?

For patients with established lymphoedema in one or more limbs, the British Lymphology Society (BLS) has developed guidelines about where to have your COVID-19 and flu vaccines. This advice, of course, applies to other vaccines as well. In short, the BLS (2023) advises:

- If you have one arm affected by lymphoedema: vaccines should be given in the unaffected, opposite arm (**Figure 2.1**).
- If you have had lymph nodes removed from the armpit of one arm: vaccines should be given in the opposite arm.
- If both arms are affected by lymphoedema, but not the legs: vaccines should be given into one of the thighs.
- If both arms and one leg are affected by lymphoedema: vaccines should be given into the unaffected thigh.
- If both arms and both legs are affected by lymphoedema: vaccines should be given into the limb least affected by lymphoedema.

## SHOULD I HAVE THE FLU, COVID-19 AND OTHER VACCINES?

You can gain immunity to a bacteria or virus by natural infection or through vaccination. The advantage of being vaccinated is that you will then be much less likely to develop the illness and then need to cope with all its complications. The very low risk of a severe complication caused by a vaccine greatly outweighs the risk of symptoms and complications caused by natural infection.

It is essential to let the doctor, nurse or pharmacist vaccinator know that you have had cancer treatment. A common question I am asked is whether it is safe to have an annual flu shot; since the pandemic, finding out about COVID-19 vaccines is also very important. The availability of and advice about vaccines for cancer patients does vary, so it's essential to check with your oncologist, haematologist, or family doctor.

If you are reading this and haven't started your cancer treatment, talk to your doctor about whether any vaccines you may need can be given before your treatment starts and your immunity drops. Many vaccines can still be given during or after treatment. Guidelines for vaccination vary from country to country, and the course you take needs to be tailored to

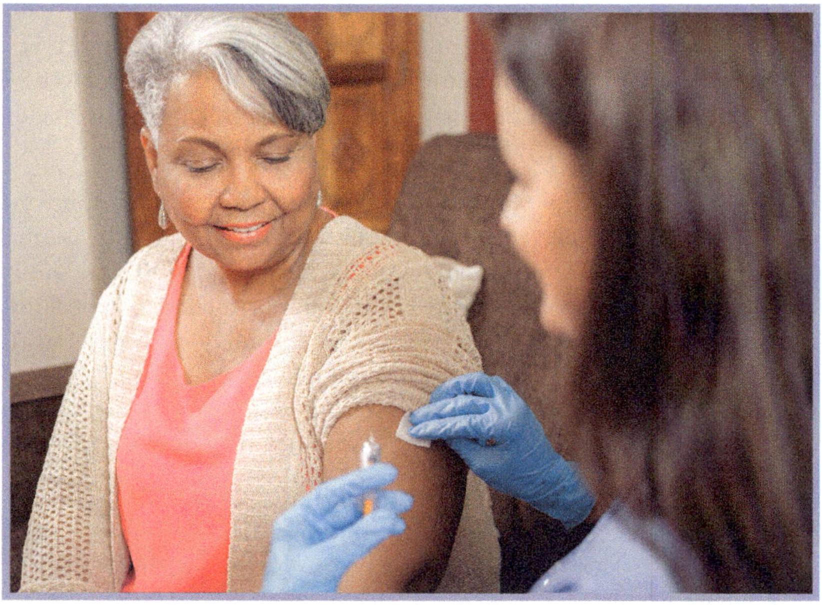

**Figure 2.1**
If you have lymphoedema or had lymph nodes removed from under your arm, request that vaccines are given in the opposite arm.

your personal situation. Factors to consider are your age, general health, past vaccination history, your occupation and the extent of your disease. Where you are up to in your cancer treatment (before, during or after) and whether the treatment has reduced your immunity is also important. I'll explain this in more detail later.

## WHEN CAN I GET MY ROUTINE VACCINES AGAIN?

The general rule is that if you have had chemotherapy and your white cell count is lower than normal, it is best to avoid live vaccines for at least three months and preferably for six months after your chemotherapy. For individual circumstances where vaccination is not considered essential, a 12-month delay may be acceptable.

If you have had radiotherapy alone, or if you are taking hormonal treatments, these are not contraindications to vaccination. It may be worthwhile having a blood count done to check that your white cell levels are back to normal. The number of white blood cells (particularly lymphocytes) may fall for a few weeks after radiation, but they usually return to normal levels by 12 months after treatment. People with breast cancer who receive radiation to the breast and lymph nodes tend to have lower lymphocyte counts than patients treated in only the breast region (Standish, 2008; Wersal, 2019).

Although these studies showed that patients had lower lymphocyte counts during treatment, they were still in the normal range. The normal lymphocyte range in adults is generally between 1,000 and 4,800 lymphocytes in one microlitre (μL) of blood, but you should check the parameters defined by the lab. As a rule of thumb, you should ensure that your lymphocyte count is within the normal range before getting vaccinated. However, influenza is a seasonal disease, and it may not be an option for some patients to wait for the vaccine until a few months after chemotherapy.

For patients undergoing or about to undergo chemotherapy, the best option may be to have the flu vaccine two weeks before starting treatment, or just before your next cycle of chemotherapy if your white blood cell counts are back to normal. Speak to your doctor about the pros and cons of getting vaccinated if you are undergoing immunotherapy, as it may trigger an increased immune response and cause side-effects.

If your **platelet** count is low, an injection may cause a nasty bruise. Again, ask your doctor about this and if you're unsure, go for a routine blood test to check your count before you have a new vaccine. If your platelets are on the low side, or if you're on blood-thinning medication, let the person doing your vaccination know this and apply pressure for at least five minutes over the injection site. This added pressure will help to stop the bleeding and prevent the formation of a **haematoma**, which is a collection of blood under the skin, similar to a bruise.

# 3

# INFLUENZA

## WHAT IS INFLUENZA?

Influenza, or 'the flu', is a **contagious** virus that infects the nose, throat and lungs and ranges from a mild disease to a severe illness causing hospitalisation or even death. Patients with cancer have reduced immunity and are at an increased risk of getting the flu and developing more complications that put them at a higher risk of dying (Pollyea, 2010).

## HOW EFFECTIVE IS THE FLU VACCINE?

The flu shot is a vaccine given to reduce your risk of catching influenza. The Cochrane centre conducted a **meta-analysis** of six studies investigating influenza vaccination in adults with cancer, three of which were randomised controlled trials (Bitterman, 2018). The studies were performed between 1993 and 2016 and featured 2,275 participants, including patients with a haematological malignancy (three studies), patients following bone marrow transplantation (two studies) and patients with a **solid malignancy** (three studies).

Two non-randomised studies showed that adults with cancer who were vaccinated had lower death rates from the flu. One small, randomised study showed a similar death rate in vaccinated and unvaccinated patients. There were significantly lower rates of influenza-like illness, pneumonia, confirmed influenza and hospitalisation for any reason among vaccine recipients in at least one study.

The Cochrane review found a weak benefit for influenza vaccination amongst adults with cancer, and the vaccine was not harmful. Influenza vaccines given to adults with cancer contain an inactivated virus that cannot cause influenza or another viral infection. The possibility for benefit shown in this review supports yearly influenza vaccination in adults with cancer who are receiving chemotherapy.

## WHY DO I NEED A FLU SHOT EVERY YEAR?

Each year, the WHO recommends which strains should be included in influenza vaccines based on global influenza epidemiology. This is because flu viruses constantly change, and the vaccine must match the circulating strains. Generally, the vaccines include at least two strains of influenza A and two of influenza B (**Figure 3.1**).

The U.S. and Australian guidelines recommend the flu vaccine for all people aged six months or older. The more potent Fluad Quad vaccine is

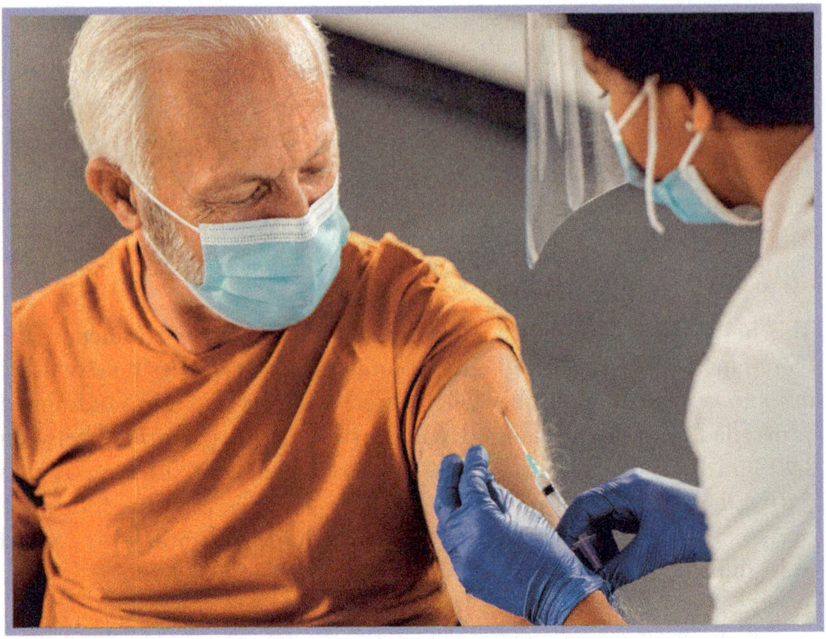

**Figure 3.1**
A man having his annual flu shot into his muscle.

advised for people who are 65 years or older. This vaccine is **adjuvanted** and includes a substance called MF59, which generates a better immune response than the standard flu vaccines (Lee, 2018).

It is best to have the inactivated (non-live) flu vaccine every year, as the strain of the virus, and therefore the composition of the vaccine, changes each year. Avoid the nasal spray flu vaccine which contains weakened live flu viruses.

## WHEN DO I HAVE MY FLU SHOT IF I AM HAVING CANCER TREATMENT?

If your doctor advises the flu vaccine during your chemotherapy treatment, have the injection on the day before your next course and ensure your white cell count has recovered to safe levels (Pollyea, 2010). There are no problems with the injectable flu vaccine if you are having radiotherapy or hormonal treatment. One study compared patients having Herceptin with those who were not and measured their immune response to the flu shot. It found no reduced immunity to the flu vaccine with the concurrent administration of Herceptin (Joona, 2020).

## CAN I HAVE MY FLU SHOT IF I'VE HAD IMMUNE CHECKPOINT INHIBITORS?

Cancer cells can produce a **checkpoint protein** to 'cloak' themselves, so the normal immune system, and particularly lymphocytes called T cells, don't recognise these abnormal cells. Immune checkpoint inhibitors (ICIs) are a type of drug that blocks the checkpoint protein, so that the T cells can better kill the now-visible cancer cells.

Patients taking ICIs should avoid live vaccines and check with their doctor before taking inactivated vaccines. ICIs include CTLA-4 inhibitors (such as ipilimumab) and PD-1 or PD-L1 inhibitors (such as nivolumab or pembrolizumab).

Some animal studies have raised concerns that ICIs may increase the body's normal immunological response against viral antigens. Part of the reason for this concern is that for patients who develop influenza or have the influenza vaccine, there is a one in a million risk of autoimmune diseases such as **Guillain-Barré syndrome** (GBS). The risk of GBS after the seasonal influenza vaccine is minimal, estimated to be between one and two additional cases per million doses. However, the CDC (2024b) believes that is it more likely for a person to contract GBS from the actual flu rather than from the vaccine.

A small study from Switzerland raised concerns that people receiving ICIs may have a higher risk of side-effects following immunisation with influenza vaccine (Laubli, 2018). However, a larger study from the Memorial Sloan Kettering Cancer Center in New York, of 370 patients over three flu seasons, found no increase in the incidence or the severity of immune-related side-effects for patients who received the flu vaccine within two months of ICIs (Chong, 2020). Notably, there were no cases of serious inflammations of the heart (myocarditis) or brain (encephalitis).

# 4

# COVID-19

## SHOULD I HAVE THE COVID-19 VACCINE?

COVID-19 vaccination remains an essential tool to protect yourself and others, especially if you have a history of cancer. While much has changed since the early days of the pandemic, vaccination continues to reduce the risk of severe illness, hospitalisation and death, even with the newer variants.

The CDC (2025b) offers the following clinical advice, last updated in May 2025:

- COVID-19 vaccination is recommended for all people aged six months and older in the United States for the prevention of COVID-19.
- Vaccination is especially important for people at higher risk of severe illness, including people aged 65 or older, people with underlying medical conditions, people living in long-term care facilities, and people who are pregnant.
- Recommended vaccines are **mRNA vaccines** (Pfizer or Moderna) or the protein subunit vaccine (Novovax); there is no preference for a specific brand, as long as the formulation is current and age-appropriate.

The Australian Technical Advisory Group on Immunisation (ATAGI) advises that people with cancer – particularly those with severe immunocompromise – receive COVID-19 vaccination every six to 12 months, depending on their age and risk (ATAGI, 2024a). In the UK, the Joint Committee on Vaccination and Immunisation similarly includes immunosuppressed people in the high-risk group eligible for seasonal COVID-19 vaccination (JCVI, 2025).

The European Society for Medical Oncology (ESMO) recommends prioritising people with cancer for ongoing COVID-19 vaccination, with a preference for mRNA vaccines (Garassino, 2021). Most European countries follow the guidance of the European Centre for Disease Prevention and Control (ECDC) to include cancer patients in national vaccination programs.

## CURRENTLY AVAILABLE COVID-19 VACCINES

It is best to check with your family doctor or pharmacist about what vaccines are available in your particular location. As of 2025, the following

COVID-19 vaccines are commonly used or approved in Australia and many other countries:

- Pfizer-BioNTech (Comirnaty) – an mRNA vaccine approved and widely used globally, including for booster doses.
- Moderna (Spikevax) – another mRNA vaccine, used for both primary and booster vaccinations.
- Novavax (Nuvaxovid) – a protein-based vaccine available in Australia for those who prefer a non-mRNA option or have contraindications to mRNA vaccines.

Some other COVID-19 vaccines include:

- AstraZeneca (Vaxzevria or Covishield) – discontinued in Australia due to rare clotting concerns but still used in some countries.
- Johnson & Johnson (Janssen) – a single-dose adenovirus vector vaccine, no longer routinely used in many countries but still authorised in some settings.

Several other vaccines exist, particularly in low- and middle-income countries:

- Sinopharm, Sinovac, and Sinopharm-Wuhan – inactivated virus vaccines developed in China.
- Covaxin – an inactivated vaccine developed in India.
- Sputnik V – a viral vector vaccine developed in Russia.

There are also updated bivalent and monovalent formulations targeting newer Omicron variants (e.g., XBB.1.5), with most countries prioritising mRNA-based vaccines for ongoing protection.

## HOW OFTEN WILL I NEED COVID-19 BOOSTER SHOTS?

Most people now require an annual COVID-19 booster, similar to the flu vaccine. However, if you have cancer or are immunocompromised you may need additional boosters every six months, depending on your treatment and immune status. mRNA vaccines (Pfizer and Moderna) are the mainstays, and updated formulations are released regularly to match circulating variants. Research has shown that boosters help restore protection against severe illness, particularly in vulnerable populations like older adults and cancer survivors.

If you've received stem-cell or CAR T-cell therapy, or are on B-cell depleting treatments, your doctor may recommend revaccination and multiple boosters to rebuild your immune response (Bar-On, 2021; Mahase, 2021; Munro, 2021). Talk to your doctor about your specific risk and the best schedule for your circumstances.

The latest Australian guidelines recommend COVID-19 booster doses every six or 12 months depending on your age and health status (ATAGI, 2024a). Adults aged 75 and over are advised to receive a dose every six months. Those aged 65 to 74 or with severe immunocompromise should have annual boosters and may consider six-monthly dosing. Others may consider vaccination based on personal risk. See **Table 4.1** for a summary of the current ATAGI recommendations.

| Age (years) | With severe immunocompromise | Without severe immunocompromise |
|---|---|---|
| <5 | Not recommended | Not recommended |
| 5–17 | Can consider every 12 months | Not recommended |
| 18–64 | Recommended every 12 months; consider a dose every 6 months | Consider a dose every 12 months |
| 65–74 | Recommended every 12 months; consider a dose every 6 months | Recommended every 12 months; consider a dose every 6 months |
| ≥ 75 | Recommended every 6 months | Recommended every 6 months |

**Table 4.1**

Timing of further COVID-19 vaccine doses by age group and risk status (ATAGI, 2024a).

## HOW EFFECTIVE ARE THE VARIOUS COVID-19 VACCINES?

Protection following two doses of a COVID-19 vaccine is initially high but declines over time. In the SIREN study of over 35,000 healthcare workers, early protection (measured 2–10 weeks after the second dose) was strongest with Pfizer: up to 89% effectiveness, dropping to 51–53% after six to eight months. AstraZeneca (AZ) started lower at 58% (Hall, 2022). Full protection develops about two weeks after the second dose of an mRNA vaccine (Pfizer or Moderna) and up to four weeks for the single-dose Johnson & Johnson (J&J) vaccine. Although the vaccines are effective, breakthrough infections can occur, especially with newer variants.

In clinical trials, Pfizer showed 95% effectiveness, Moderna 94%, Novavax 89%, and AZ around 70%. The AZ vaccine's effectiveness increased to 80% if the second dose was delayed until 12 weeks after the first dose, but fell to 60% when given sooner (Voysey, 2021a, 2021b). J&J showed 66% protection against symptomatic COVID-19 and 100% protection against hospitalisation and death. In real-world UK data, both Pfizer and AZ provided over 95% protection against hospitalisation and death (Lopez Bernal, 2021).

While vaccinated individuals can still get COVID-19, especially with the newer variants, they tend to have milder symptoms and are less likely to transmit the virus. Booster doses are recommended for older adults and people with weakened immunity to maintain protection.

## COVID-19 VACCINE AFTER BEING INFECTED WITH COVID-19

Different countries recommend slightly different timing for vaccination after a COVID-19 infection. In Australia, vaccination is generally advised six months (180 days) after infection. In the U.S., the CDC recommends waiting at least three months, while the UK advises waiting about four weeks (28 days) if symptoms have resolved (Hall, 2022).

In the SIREN study, people who had COVID-19 previously and then got vaccinated (known as 'hybrid immunity') had the best and most durable protection – over 90% – even after a year, regardless of how long after their infection they received the vaccine. The timing between the first and second vaccine dose did not make a big difference, with longer intervals (six weeks or more) being just as effective as shorter intervals.

## CAN I HAVE THE COVID-19 VACCINE DURING MY CHEMOTHERAPY?

Yes, you can receive the COVID-19 vaccine during chemotherapy, and current guidelines recommend doing so as soon as possible rather than delaying. The CDC, ATAGI and ESMO all advise prioritising vaccination for people undergoing cancer treatment, including chemotherapy, without needing to time it around the treatment cycles.

While the optimal window during chemotherapy treatment remains unclear, most experts agree that delaying vaccination may pose a greater risk, especially during a period of high community transmission. One practical approach is to schedule the vaccine a day or two before your next cycle of chemotherapy, when your white cell counts may be higher. A French study found that only 48% of patients undergoing chemotherapy developed detectable antibodies four weeks after their first Pfizer dose, compared to 77% in cancer patients not on chemotherapy and 100% in healthy control participants (Barrière, 2021). However, by eight weeks, 95% of chemotherapy patients had developed COVID-19 antibodies, suggesting a strong immune response after the second dose. This reinforces the importance of receiving both doses on schedule and not delaying booster vaccines.

While on chemotherapy, you should still take precautions (e.g., masking, social distancing) after vaccination due to the risk of a reduced or impaired immune response to the vaccine. Likewise, your close contacts should be fully vaccinated and continue taking precautions to help protect you and any other immunocompromised individuals.

## CAN I HAVE THE COVID-19 VACCINE WHILE ON IMMUNOTHERAPY?

You should discuss the decision to have the vaccine with your treatment team if you are receiving immunotherapy treatment such as atezolizumab, which is sometimes used for advanced triple-negative breast cancer. In a study from Israel, cancer patients being treated with immune checkpoint inhibitors (mainly pembrolizumab and nivolumab) who received the Pfizer vaccine did not experience any more side-effects than patients without cancer. Most importantly, no new side-effects or worsening of existing immune-related side-effects were observed (Waissengrin, 2021).

## CAN I HAVE THE COVID-19 VACCINE DURING RADIATION THERAPY?

Yes. All currently available COVID-19 vaccines are inactivated (non-live) vaccines and are considered safe during radiation therapy. The American Society for Radiation Oncology advises that patients actively receiving treatment discuss the timing and location (injection site) of the vaccine with their radiation oncologist, particularly if their radiation treatment involves lymph nodes, as any swelling could be misinterpreted (ASTRO, 2021).

In the UK, it is recommended that people undergoing cancer treatment, including radiation therapy, should be vaccinated as soon as possible, without needing to delay either treatment or vaccination (Cancer Research UK, 2025). In Australia, ATAGI (2025a) also supports vaccination during cancer treatment, including radiation, with no specific contraindications or schedule changes required.

Although minor side-effects such as fatigue or fever may overlap with treatment symptoms, spacing the vaccine a day or two from your radiation session may help avoid confusion. Individuals not currently undergoing active treatment can receive the vaccine whenever eligible.

## CAN I HAVE THE COVID-19 VACCINE WHILE ON HORMONAL TREATMENT OR HERCEPTIN?

Yes. Hormone therapies commonly used in breast cancer, such as tamoxifen, letrozole, anastrozole, and exemestane, do not significantly affect the immune system. Similarly, anti-HER2 treatments like Herceptin (trastuzumab) are not immunosuppressive, so it is safe to receive the COVID-19 vaccine while undergoing these therapies.

Patients with prostate cancer receiving hormone therapy, including anti-androgens, can also be vaccinated without concerns about reduced vaccine effectiveness.

## IS THE COVID-19 VACCINE SAFE IF I HAVE ALLERGIES?

The vaccine is safe for most people with common allergies such as hay fever, food allergies, or insect stings. However, if you have a history of anaphylaxis or multiple drug allergies – particularly to drugs containing polyethylene glycol (PEG) or polysorbate 80 – you should consult an allergist or immunologist. They may recommend skin-prick testing or supervised vaccination in a medical setting.

Vaccine-related anaphylaxis is extremely rare, usually occurring within 20 to 30 minutes, and most cases respond well to one or two doses of adrenaline (epinephrine). If you are concerned, consider being vaccinated at a hospital-based clinic or larger medical centre rather than a small pharmacy or GP office.

The Australian Immunisation Handbook (ATAGI, 2025a) advises avoiding COVID-19 vaccines only if:

- you have had anaphylaxis to a previous dose of a COVID-19 vaccine, or
- you have had anaphylaxis to a known ingredient, such as PEG (Pfizer) or polysorbate 80 (AstraZeneca).

If you are unwell (e.g., if you have flu-like symptoms), delay vaccination and consider a COVID-19 test first.

## WHAT IS THE RISK OF BLOOD CLOTS AFTER THE COVID-19 VACCINE?

In 2021, rare cases of blood clots with low platelet counts (called **thrombosis** with **thrombocytopenia** syndrome, or TTS) were reported after vaccination with the J&J and AZ vaccines. These cases were mostly in younger women and occurred within two weeks of vaccination.

Health authorities in the U.S. and UK temporarily paused the use of these vaccines while they investigated. Use later resumed with added warnings for younger age groups. TTS was a very rare side-effect and has become even less common as these vaccines are now rarely used in most countries. mRNA vaccines (like Pfizer and Moderna) have not been linked to this syndrome.

## WHAT IS THE RISK OF HEART COMPLICATIONS AFTER THE COVID-19 VACCINE?

In June 2021, *JAMA Cardiology* featured two case series describing a rare complication of mRNA-based COVID-19 vaccines called myocarditis, or inflammation of the heart (Shay, 2021).

In the first report from Duke University, three cases occurred in men aged 23 to 36 years and the fourth in a 70-year-old woman (Kim, 2021). All four patients had received the second dose of an mRNA vaccine (two Moderna and two Pfizer vaccines). All cases presented one to five days after having had the second dose of their COVID-19 vaccine. All presented with sudden, severe chest pain. They had an abnormal electrocardiogram (ECG) and evidence of heart damage as shown by increased troponin levels in their blood test. A magnetic resonance imaging (MRI) scan confirmed the diagnosis.

The second report from the military health system described 23 individuals who experienced sudden myocarditis. Again, they presented within four days of their second dose of an mRNA-based COVID-19 vaccine (Montgomery, 2021). Sixteen of these patients received the Moderna vaccine and seven had the Pfizer vaccine. Twenty of the 23 developed myocarditis after the second dose of the vaccine. The three patients presenting after their first vaccine dose had COVID-19 infection more than two months before vaccination.

This type of immune reaction to the heart was previously described after smallpox vaccination. In the Duke series, the estimated incidence of myocarditis was 1 in 140,000. The military health system estimated a risk of 1 in 23,000 active-duty military men. The most comprehensive data from Israel estimated a risk of 1 in 46,000 vaccinated among younger men aged 16 to 19 years, usually after the second dose. Most cases have been in the hospital for up to four days, and 95% are considered mild cases.

It's important to seek urgent medical advice if you have any of these symptoms within a few days of being vaccinated:

- chest pain
- shortness of breath
- a fast-beating, fluttering, or pounding heart (palpitations).

## WHAT IS MY RISK OF DYING IF I CONTRACT COVID-19?

As we have seen in countries such as India, USA and Brazil, it is easy for COVID-19 to get out of control. The higher the incidence of disease, the higher the number of admissions to hospital and subsequent increases in intensive care unit (ICU) admission and death. We saw the enormous pressure on hospital systems in Italy at the start of the pandemic in early 2020, and the dire situation in India in May 2021. The risk of dying from COVID-19 increases if you are older, overweight, male or have other chronic illnesses. The risk is also higher for patients with active cancer (i.e., not in remission). Some studies found a higher death rate among patients with cancer who were diagnosed with COVID-19 while on active treatment – and not just the patients having chemotherapy (Kuderer, 2020). The overall death rate 30 days after a diagnosis of COVID-19 was 13%. Notably, it was exceptionally high for patients with active and progressive cancer: 22% for those with non-haematological (solid) tumours and 25% for those with haematological cancers.

Depending on the country you live in and the background incidence of COVID-19, it is also important to get vaccinated if you have had cancer in the past. For patients in remission, death rates from COVID-19 were lower: 10% for people with previous solid cancers and 12% for haematological cancers (Kuderer, 2020).

## COMPARING THE RISK OF DYING FROM THE COVID-19 VACCINE TO OTHER RISKS

So, back to some good news: the risk of dying from a COVID-19 vaccine is extremely low – around one in a million based on UK data, and even lower in Australia, where it's estimated to be closer to one in two million. To put this in perspective, the risk is far less than many of the everyday risks we accept, such as driving in city traffic, flying in an aeroplane, or even catching the flu.

While cases of serious blood clots such as TTS were initially reported with adenoviral vaccines like AZ and J&J, these vaccines are now rarely used. Importantly, Australia's lower death rate from vaccine-related clots likely reflects early detection, prompt treatment, and careful rollout to appropriate age groups.

Ultimately, we must weigh this incredibly small vaccine risk against the much higher risks posed by COVID-19 itself – especially for older adults and people with cancer. These include hospitalisation, long COVID, and the social impact of lockdowns, delays in treatment, and travel restrictions. When viewed in context, vaccination remains the far safer choice.

# Mitra's Story

I'm 60 years old and was previously in very good health. Then, just before Christmas 2020, I noticed a firmness in my left breast. Soon afterwards, I was diagnosed with two breast cancers, both high-grade hormone-positive tumours. One was positive for HER2 while the other was negative.

I received neoadjuvant chemotherapy consisting of dose-dense AC followed by Taxol and HER2-targeted therapy drugs. This treatment was extremely challenging, and I experienced fungal pneumonia due to chemo-induced neutropenia, as well as tachycardia and shortness of breath. I was admitted to hospital for overnight stays on several occasions. Despite all these challenges, I was able to have my lumpectomy, followed by a successful revision surgery, in July 2021. The cancer had largely disappeared after my chemo.

The second wave of the COVID-19 outbreak took hold in Sydney in June 2021. I was nervous about receiving the COVID-19 vaccine given my complications, but I also knew I needed protection given all the treatments I had received. In addition, I was also about to start radiotherapy.

I received my first dose of the Pfizer vaccine, and three days afterwards, I started experiencing shortness of breath and tightness and pains in my chest. My GP ordered blood tests (troponin and creatine kinase), which showed I was experiencing myocarditis. I was admitted to hospital and spent a night in the coronary care unit. When discharged, I was ordered to rest at home and get my blood troponin level checked every week. My symptoms are now improving, although my blood troponin level is still elevated.

Obviously, I know I need to be fully vaccinated, and at the time of writing I am due for my second shot. However, I'm still waiting for definitive advice from my doctors regarding when I can have it. My oncologist has consulted experts who agreed with his suggestion that instead of having a second Pfizer, I should now receive two doses of the AstraZeneca vaccine, 12 weeks apart. The third dose will act as a booster given my reduced immunity.

# 5

# SHINGLES

## WHAT IS SHINGLES?

The varicella zoster virus causes chickenpox (varicella) in children and can reappear later in life as **shingles (zoster)**. After a chickenpox infection – or even after vaccination – the virus stays dormant in nerve clusters near the spine. It can reactivate decades later. Most cases of shingles occur in people over 50, who carry the highest risk of reactivation and complications.

In adults, shingles can cause quite a lot of pain and a severe rash, as well as serious complications. Common locations for shingles are the chest area, the face, and the eye. The rash can be serious if it spreads across your eye and may require hospital admission. An early sign of zoster affecting the face and eye may be a rash on the tip, side and root of the nose, known as Hutchinson's sign (Sampathkumar, 2009).

Symptoms can be more severe in cancer patients who have reduced immunity after radiation and/or chemotherapy. The rash consists of blisters that usually crust over in seven to 10 days and clear up within two to four weeks. The pain can be intense and burning. It can last for months or even years after the rash goes away. This long-lasting pain is called **postherpetic neuralgia**, the most common complication of shingles (**Figure 5.1**).

## HOW IS SHINGLES DIAGNOSED?

Early detection and treatment of shingles can reduce the severity of the initial symptoms and may also reduce postherpetic neuralgia. Warning symptoms include itching, a painful burning, prickling or achiness and pain along the distribution of the involved **dermatome** (see Janet's story, page 15).

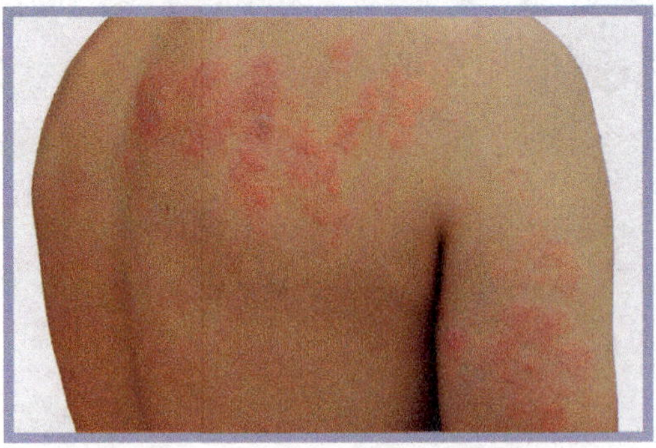

**Figure 5.1**

A shingles rash looks like a large cold sore and may weep and feel painful and itchy. It eventually scabs over and heals. Note that it does not extend beyond the mid-line of the back.

A dermatome is a patch of skin whose sensation comes from a single nerve from the spine. These types of unusual symptoms at the dermatome may occur several days before the rash appears. The pain can sometimes be mistaken for other conditions such as colic, heart attack, dental pain, or pleurisy, leading to a delay in diagnosis. A swab can be taken to formally diagnose shingles in the lab.

## HOW COMMON IS SHINGLES?

The lifetime risk of shingles is estimated to be about 30% (Brisson, 2001). The Australian Institute of Health and Welfare notes that it is most common in those aged over 50. In 2022, there were 2,412 hospital admissions for shingles in Australia and 65 deaths (AIHW, 2025).

In the U.S., it is estimated that one million people develop shingles each year. The incidence increases with age, from five cases per 1,000 population in adults aged 50–59 years to 11 cases per 1,000 population in persons aged 80 years or over (Dooling, 2018).

Cancer patients have a higher overall incidence of shingles compared with age-matched controls. A large UK study of about 200,000 adult patients with shingles found that a previous cancer diagnosis was associated with a small but clear increase in the chance of shingles (Hansson, 2017). The highest risk of shingles was associated with haematological malignancies (blood cancer): for patients with lymphoma and leukaemia, the chance of getting shingles was more than doubled, and myeloma was associated with a quadrupling of the risk. For solid cancers (i.e., non-haematological), the increase in the risk of contracting zoster was greatest for brain cancer. Oral, oesophageal, stomach, colorectal, lung, breast, ovarian, prostate, kidney and bladder cancers were also associated with a smaller increase.

This association between cancer and zoster was larger among younger patients, and the risk typically peaked within three years after diagnosis. The authors argued that vaccination to prevent shingles should be strongly considered as soon as possible after diagnosis or treatment of cancer.

## IS SHINGLES CONTAGIOUS?

The problem with the shingles rash is that it contains high concentrations of the zoster virus, which can be spread by contact and the airborne route and can cause chickenpox in previously unexposed, susceptible persons.

It is not as infectious as chickenpox and is only contagious after the rash appears and until the lesions crust over. The risk of transmission is reduced if the lesions are covered.

## WHAT VACCINES ARE AVAILABLE FOR SHINGLES?

In Australia, the shingles vaccine is recommended for all people aged 50 years and over, and people 18 years and over who are immunocompromised (ATAGI, 2025g). Vaccination is funded by the National Immunisation Program (NIP) for older adults and selected groups with moderate or severe immunocompromise; other people may need to pay privately.

The first shingles vaccine was Zostavax®, a live attenuated vaccine that came out in 2006. A randomised trial found that the efficacy of Zostavax was 64% for those aged 60–69 years, and 38% in people aged 70 or over, with an average follow-up time of three years. The efficacy against postherpetic neuralgia was about two-thirds (66%) for both age groups (Dooling, 2018). The effectiveness of the vaccine reduced over time.

A newer vaccine, Shingrix®, was released in 2017. In 2023 it replaced Zostavax on the NIP. A free two-dose course of Shingrix is now offered in Australia to adults from age 65, Aboriginal and Torres Strait Islander adults from age 50, and selected groups of immunocompromised people from age 18 (ATAGI, 2025g). This includes most patients receiving chemotherapy, targeted therapy and immunotherapy, and those with haematological malignancies (ATAGI, 2024b).

Shingrix is now the main shingles vaccine available around the world. Shingrix is preferred because it is an inactivated vaccine. It is given in two doses administered into the muscle, two to six months apart.

As a non-live vaccine, Shingrix can be given to patients with cancer, even if they are receiving or have recently received radiation or chemotherapy. It was originally tested on adult patients who had solid tumours and were receiving chemotherapy (López-Fauqued, 2021; Vink, 2019).

The efficacy of Shingrix was evaluated in a clinical trial of more than 30,000 participants who randomly received either the vaccine or a saline **placebo**. The follow-up period was about three-and-a-half years. The efficacy was approximately 97% for ages up to 69 and 91% for 70 years or over. In people aged 70 or over, vaccine efficacy was 98% in the first year after vaccination and 85% or higher for the remaining three years of the study. Efficacy for the prevention of postherpetic neuralgia was about

90%. In other words, Shingrix was far more effective and safer than the Zostavax live vaccine.

Shingrix was also tested in close to 2,000 bone marrow transplant patients, with the first dose given 50 to 70 days after transplantation, and then a booster dose one to two months later. During the 21-month median follow-up, at least one episode of shingles was confirmed in 49 vaccine and 135 placebo recipients, equivalent to 68.2% vaccine efficacy (Bastidas, 2019). For patients with solid tumours, the initial immune response was higher if Shingrix was given before rather than during chemotherapy, but responses were similar 12 months after vaccination (Vink, 2019).

Shingrix is given into the muscle. Significant injection-site reactions (pain, redness and swelling) were reported in about 10% (100 in 1,000) of recipients compared to 0.3% (3 in 1,000) of the placebo group. Significant generalised reactions, such as muscle pain, fatigue, headache, shivering, fever, and gastrointestinal symptoms, were reported by about 10% of vaccine recipients and 2% of placebo recipients. Side-effects usually resolve within three days. Generalised reactions were reported more frequently after the second dose of the vaccine.

## WHAT PRECAUTIONS SHOULD I TAKE IF I GET SHINGLES?

If you are unlucky enough to get shingles, it is important to take precautions to protect the people around you:

- Cover the rash (if possible).
- Avoid touching or scratching the rash.
- Wash your hands often to prevent the virus from spreading.
- Avoid contact with the following groups of people until your rash has developed crusts:
  - pregnant women who have never had chickenpox or the chickenpox vaccine
  - premature or low-birthweight babies
  - children who have not had chickenpox or the chickenpox vaccine
  - people with weakened immune systems, e.g., people having chemotherapy or taking immunosuppressive medication; transplant recipients; and people living with human immunodeficiency virus (HIV).

**See https://www.healthdirect.gov.au/shingles for more information.**

Your risk of developing postherpetic neuralgia decreases if you begin taking antiviral medications within 72 hours of developing the shingles rash. See your doctor urgently if you get an unusual, itchy rash on one side of your body. Antiviral medicines include famciclovir (250 mg, three times daily for seven days), valaciclovir (1 g, three times daily for seven days) or aciclovir (800 mg, five times daily for seven days).

## SHOULD I HAVE THE SHINGLES VACCINE?

If you've had cancer treatment, or are about to start, you should seriously think about protecting yourself against shingles. Shingrix is recommended in Australia, the U.S. and the UK for adults aged 18 and over who have a weakened immune system, or are expected to have one soon—and this includes most people having cancer treatment. Shingrix can be given at any time before, during, or after your cancer treatment (see **Table 11.1**).

## Janet's Story

I'm 69 years old and found a lump that was biopsied just before Christmas 2020. On New Year's Eve, I was told I had breast cancer. It was awful waiting for the results at that time of the year. The cancer was small, but high grade. I had a lumpectomy and a sentinel node biopsy.

I developed an itchy spot in the upper part of my left breast. I'd just finished four courses of chemotherapy and was about to start my radiation. The spot became itchy and developed some watery bubbles. I tried cortisone cream, but that didn't help, and the rash kept spreading across the top part of my breast. I then tried an antiseptic cream over the weekend and went and saw my general practitioner on the Tuesday.

My general practitioner diagnosed herpes zoster (shingles), took a swab, and started me on Valtrex. This began to soothe the rash, and the spot started to crust over. I called my radiation team who decided to delay the start of my radiation by one week as the rash was in the treatment area. The rash seems to have scarred my skin and I'm hoping this will improve. Once it had scabbed over and wasn't weeping anymore, my radiation team started my treatment.

A good friend of mine developed bad shingles across her eye and I know how bad it can get. My husband hasn't had his zoster vaccine either. My general practitioner told me that the vaccine is given after the age of 70 in Australia. However, my chemotherapy had reduced my immunity and reactivated the chickenpox virus I had had as a child. I'm lucky my case wasn't as bad as my friend's shingles.

# 6

# PNEUMOCOCCAL DISEASE

## WHAT IS PNEUMOCOCCAL DISEASE?

Pneumococcus (*Streptococcus pneumoniae*) infection may have serious implications for patients with cancer. It can cause sinus and middle ear infections, pneumonia, blood poisoning, serious bone or joint infections or meningitis. The more serious form of the infection is known as invasive pneumococcal disease (IPD). The incidence and risk of dying from IPD increases with age (**Table 6.1**).

| Age (years) | Disease incidence (IPD cases per million) | Mortality rate (IPD deaths per million) | Case fatality ratio* (%) |
|---|---|---|---|
| 5–17 | 23 | 1 | 4.3 |
| 18–34 | 31 | 2 | 6.5 |
| 35–49 | 74 | 6 | 8.1 |
| 50–64 | 132 | 18 | 13.6 |
| 65–74 | 158 | 17 | 10.8 |
| 75–84 | 164 | 27 | 16.5 |
| ≥85 | 274 | 75 | 27.4 |
| Total | 83 | 10 | 12.0 |

* Case fatality ratio [(total deaths ÷ total cases)×100] estimates the risk of dying if you are diagnosed with the disease.

**Table 6.1**

Risk of developing and dying from serious invasive pneumococcal disease (IPD) in 2022 by age (Gierke, 2025).

The data above comes from ongoing surveillance of *S. pneumoniae* in the United States by the CDC. Approximately 12% of patients who develop IPD will die from the disease, but this rate is impacted by age and other health conditions. Pneumococcus infection leads to a number of different diseases, presenting most commonly as ear infections in children and as pneumonia in adults. Although non-invasive disease is harder to measure, approximately two million pneumococcal infections occur each year in the U.S., causing 6,000 deaths (Gierke, 2025).

## HOW CURRENT IS PNEUMOCOCCAL DISEASE AFTER CANCER?

The disease rates for adults with cancer who have reduced immunity can be more than 20 times higher than adults without high-risk medical conditions (Bennett, 2012). In 2010, the incidence of IPD in people aged 18 to 64 with blood cancer (haematological malignancies) was 19% – four times higher than the risk for elderly people over 85 without cancer. A Canadian study found that patients undergoing chemotherapy for solid tumours had a risk of IPD up to 50 times higher than that of healthy adults, with death rates approaching 35% (Shigayeva, 2016).

## TYPES OF PNEUMOCOCCAL VACCINE

There are two types of pneumococcal vaccines:

- The pneumococcal **polysaccharide vaccine** contains polysaccharides (sugar) from the capsule of pneumococcal bacteria. PPSV23 (also called PPV, 23vPPV or Pneumovax 23®) contains polysaccharides from 23 different strains of *S. pneumoniae.* PPSV23 is used around the world, but mainly for adults, as it has limited effectiveness in children.
- Pneumococcal **conjugate vaccines** contain polysaccharides that are chemically linked (conjugated) to a protein, enhancing the body's ability to develop a strong and lasting immune response. They include:
  - PCV13 (13vPCV or Prevenar/Prevnar 13®)
  - PCV15 (15vPCV or Vaxneuvance®)
  - PCV20 (20vPCV or Prevenar/Prevnar 20®)

All pneumococcal vaccines are inactivated, and they are injected into the muscle. PPSV23 can be given under the skin, but this increases the reaction at the injection site.

## HOW EFFECTIVE IS THE PNEUMOCOCCAL VACCINE?

In one trial, a single dose of PCV13 was compared to PPSV23 in 831 patients who were previously unvaccinated for pneumococcal disease. PCV13 achieved a stronger immune response than PPSV23 for most of the strains covered by PCV13 (Jackson, 2013).

In a clinical trial known as 'CAPiTA' (community-acquired pneumonia immunization trial in adults), the efficacy of PCV13 in adults aged 65 years or older against community-acquired pneumonia was 46%, and against IPD was 75%. All vaccinated participants, even the elderly, showed a strong immune response to the vaccine, developing antibodies against the 13 serotypes at significantly higher levels than baseline, and consistently higher than the placebo group, over the two years of the trial (van Deursen, 2017). A subsequent study in patients with Hodgkin lymphoma showed that giving a conjugated vaccine (PCV7), followed by PPSV23 one year later, resulted in a much better immune response (Seth, 2025).

An Australian study found that starting a routine vaccination program for people who had received a bone marrow transplant caused the number of IPD infections to drop dramatically, from around 40 cases per 1,000 people to just four per 1,000 (Roberts, 2020). Other studies have shown that people with certain cancers – such as multiple myeloma, chronic lymphocytic leukaemia, stomach cancer and bowel cancer – can still make a good immune response to the vaccine. In more than half of these patients, their blood showed a strong antibody response after vaccination, even if they had undergone a bone marrow transplant (Garcia Garrido, 2021).

Newer pneumococcal vaccines have been tested in adults and found to be safe and effective. PCV15 produces equal or better protection compared to older vaccines, and PCV20 protects against more strains of the pneumococcus bacteria. PCV21 (Capvaxive®), the most recent version, covers even more strains and has been shown to work well in older people and those with weaker immune systems. These vaccines are now recommended in the U.S. as a simple, one-dose option for adults at higher risk, including people with cancer. Other countries, including Australia, are reviewing their use (El-Beyrouty, 2022; Kobayashi, 2024).

**The pneumococcal vaccination program in Australia is under review at the time of writing. For the latest updates, refer to the Australian Immunisation Handbook (immunisationhandbook.health.gov.au) or talk to your GP.**

## TIMING OF THE PNEUMOCOCCAL VACCINE

The pneumococcal vaccine is available at any time of the year. The recommended interval between the dose of PCV13 and the first dose of PPSV23 is 12 months, although a gap of at least two months is acceptable. The recommended interval between the two PPSV23 doses is at least five years.

In Australia, the latest guidelines recommend that adults newly diagnosed with cancer receive one dose of PCV13 (Prevenar 13) followed by two doses of PPSV23 (Pneumovax 23). The first dose of PPSV23 should be administered 12 months (or a minimum of two months) after PCV13, and the second should be given at least five years later.

PCV13 and PPSV23 are funded under the NIP for people with haematological malignancies, those who have had a bone marrow transplant, and all adults aged 70 years or older. Although PCV15 and PCV20 are approved by the Therapeutic Goods Administration (TGA) and registered for adult use in Australia, they are still under review for inclusion in the NIP. Consequently, they are not currently funded for immunocompromised adults.

PCV20 has recently been added to the NIP for young people in Australia. From 1 September 2025, Prevenar 20 replaces both Prevenar 13 and Pneumovax 23 on the immunisation schedule for children and adolescents. The adult schedule remains unchanged (Department of Health, Disability and Ageing, 2025).

Current U.S. guidelines (CDC, 2024c) recommend that adults aged 19 years or older with immunocompromising conditions, including cancer, receive one of the following:

- a single dose of PCV20 or PCV21 (these vaccines provide broad protection, so follow-up doses are not required)
- one dose of PCV15 followed by a dose of PPSV23 at least eight weeks later.

If PPSV23 was given first, a dose of PCV15, PCV20, or PCV21 should be administered at least one year later. If the person previously received PCV13, then a single dose of PCV20 or PCV21 should be given at least one year after the PCV13 dose; no further pneumococcal vaccines are needed, regardless of whether PCV20 or PCV21 is used.

A second dose of PPSV23 is only recommended if the first PPSV23 dose was given before age 65, and at least five years have passed since that dose.

## WHAT ARE THE SIDE-EFFECTS OF THE PNEUMOCOCCAL VACCINE?

The pneumococcal vaccine is generally safe and well tolerated. In adults, it can be given at the same time other vaccines for shingles, flu, RSV and COVID-19 if required (ATAGI, 2025c).

The most common side-effects of both PCV13 and PPSV23 include redness, pain, swelling, or warmth at the injection site. Some people also experience tiredness, headache, chills, reduced appetite, or mild muscle aches. These reactions are usually mild and settle within a couple of days. Like any vaccine, it should not be given to anyone with a severe allergic reaction to a previous dose or to any of its components – such as CRM197, which is a type of deactivated diphtheria toxin used as a carrier protein in some conjugate vaccines.

## SHOULD I HAVE THE PNEUMOCOCCAL VACCINE?

Yes – if your immune system has been weakened by cancer treatment such as chemotherapy, it's a good idea to have the pneumococcal vaccine. It helps protect you against serious infections, especially when your body's defences are low. Ideally, the vaccine should be given before you start chemotherapy or at least three months after your treatment is completed. If you have undergone very intensive treatments, like those for leukaemia, waiting at least six months is recommended.

In the past, people with weakened immunity were advised to have PCV13, followed by PPSV23 eight weeks later. Today, newer vaccines like PCV20 and PCV21 are available in some countries and may be used as a single-dose option in high-risk adults.

# 7

# WHOOPING COUGH

## WHAT IS WHOOPING COUGH (PERTUSSIS)?

Pertussis is known as whooping (pronounced as in 'hoop') cough because of the sound that someone makes when gasping for air after a fit of coughing. Pertussis is potentially dangerous for babies, as they cannot get vaccinated until they are at least six weeks old.

Serious but rare complications can occur, including middle ear infections, chronic bronchitis, pneumonia, encephalopathy (inflammation of the brain), rib fractures, a collapsed lung or bleeding around the brain. The risk of severe complications and death is highest in infants under six months. Therefore, it is important for adults around babies to be vaccinated against whooping cough.

Coughing fits due to pertussis infection can last up to 10 weeks or more (also known as the '100-day cough') and about 50% of babies who get pertussis end up in hospital.

## THE WHOOPING COUGH VACCINE

The CDC (2024d) advises that the most effective way to prevent pertussis is through vaccination with a combined diphtheria, tetanus and pertussis vaccine: DTaP for babies and children and Tdap for preteens, teens, and adults.

- Vaccination of pregnant women is especially important to help protect babies.
- Vaccinated children and adults can become infected with pertussis and infect others; however, the disease is typically much less severe in vaccinated people.
- Clinicians generally treat pertussis with antibiotics to control symptoms and spread of the disease.

Pertussis vaccine is only available in Australia and many other countries in combination with diphtheria and tetanus. Vaccines may also include inactivated poliovirus, hepatitis B and *Haemophilus influenzae* type b (Hib). The acronym names vary: diphtheria, tetanus, and acellular pertussis-containing vaccines are called 'DTPa' and 'dTpa' in Australia, while other countries use 'DTaP' and 'Tdap'. (It doesn't matter what order the letters are in, as long as upper/lower case is correct.) The capital letters in DTPa signify the higher dose used in child formulations. The lower-case dTpa means the vaccine contains substantially fewer diphtheria toxoid and pertussis antigens than the child formulation. My wife and I had the Boostrix® dTpa combination vaccine when our grandson Jack was born in 2013 and our granddaughter Elsie in 2020.

To protect newborns from whooping cough, make sure pregnant people receive a dTpa vaccine during each pregnancy. Grandparents or other carers who have not already had a whooping cough booster should also be vaccinated. If a teen or adult will be in close contact with the baby and has already had a dTpa vaccine, they do not need to be vaccinated again.

## TREATMENT FOR WHOOPING COUGH

Patients with suspected or known pertussis should start antibiotics as soon as possible to prevent disease spread. If antibiotics are started during the first phase, known as the catarrhal phase, the symptoms may be fewer and of shorter duration. This first phase includes symptoms such as a runny nose, mild cough, and red eyes. Antibiotics will help prevent the further spread of infection to susceptible contacts. All close and household contacts should receive preventative treatment (**prophylaxis**) with antibiotics.

Antibiotics known as macrolides (e.g., azithromycin, erythromycin) are recommended for both treatment and prophylaxis of pertussis. Azithromycin is the drug of choice for all age groups. For patients who are unable to tolerate, or are allergic to, the macrolide class of antibiotics, trimethoprim/sulfamethoxazole (Bactrim®) is the alternative drug that may be used in all age groups.

## SHOULD I BE VACCINATED FOR WHOOPING COUGH?

The CDC recommends whooping cough vaccines for people of all ages. A small study from the Memorial Sloane Kettering Cancer Center found that cancer patients with compromised immunity are potentially at an increased risk of acquiring pertussis due to the accelerated loss of immunity during cancer treatment (Robilotti, 2020).

This loss of immunity is most well established for recipients of bone marrow transplants and children undergoing intensive forms of chemotherapy. The study concluded that overcoming barriers and missed opportunities to vaccinate patients following a bone marrow transplant, and prioritising at-risk populations within the oncology setting, would further help to prevent pertussis.

**If you're visiting a newborn and haven't had a booster in the past 10 years, ask your GP about a dTpa shot.**

All patients should be up to date on tetanus and diphtheria toxoid (dT or Td) immunisation. Adults who have never received a dTpa vaccine, or who had the vaccine more than 10 years ago, should be vaccinated (**Table 11.1**).

# 8

# Q FEVER

## WHAT IS Q FEVER?

Q fever was first recognised as a human disease at a meat plant in Brisbane, Australia in 1937 (Eldin, 2017). The 'Q' stands for 'query' and was assigned when the cause was unknown. Q fever is now known to be caused by the bacteria *Coxiella burnetii.*

Q fever is a public health concern in many countries, including France, the UK, Italy, Spain, Germany, Israel, Greece, and Canada (Maurin, 1999). A large outbreak occurred in the Netherlands between 2007 and 2010, when over 4,000 cases were reported (Schneeberger, 2014).

In Australia, *C. burnetii* is present in rural areas in kangaroos, bandicoots, rodents and associated ticks. The ticks then infect feral and domestic goats, cattle, or sheep. Within Australia, most cases occur in Queensland, followed by New South Wales. Transmission to humans is usually due to breathing in dust contaminated with infected animal body fluids. Human-to-human transmission does not generally occur.

## WHO IS AT RISK OF Q FEVER?

People in direct or indirect contact with animals are at risk. The Q fever bug can survive for long periods in the environment, even in the harshest of conditions, and may be carried long distances in the air by the wind. Q fever can also survive in soil and dust, and infect animal products and materials such as clothing and straw.

The Australian Immunisation Handbook (ATAGI, 2025d) lists the following groups as being at high risk of contracting Q fever:

- abattoir workers
- farmers
- stockyard workers
- shearers
- animal transporters
- veterinarians, vet nurses and vet students
- professional dog and cat breeders
- pet food manufacturing workers
- agricultural college staff and students
- wildlife and zoo staff who work with high-risk animals

- animal refuge workers
- laboratory workers who handle veterinary specimens or work with *C. burnetii*
- people who cull or process kangaroos or camels
- other people exposed to high-risk animals.

## WHAT ARE THE SYMPTOMS OF Q FEVER?

Q fever may present as a flu-like illness. Most infected people develop fever, headaches (often described as being behind the eyes), muscle pain, lethargy, coughing and night sweats. In acute Q fever, the fever occurs abruptly, reaches as high as 40°C and can last more than 15 days (Eldin, 2017). Cases may either be mild or have no symptoms. Pneumonia occurs in two out of three infected people, and hepatitis occurs in about one in six people. Inflammation of the lining of the brain or heart rarely occurs.

Approximately one to five per cent of cases can progress to chronic Q fever. Common manifestations of this include inflammation of the heart valves (endocarditis), infection of blood vessels (vascular infections) for patients with pre-existing aneurysms or vascular grafts, and infection within artificial joints (prostheses). Arthritis, osteomyelitis and hepatitis can occur, but are very rare. Some patients lose weight with chronic Q fever but the disease is rarely fatal. A post-infection fatigue syndrome (sometimes labeled as chronic fatigue syndrome) can occur in up to one in five patients.

A two-week course of antibiotic tablets is generally used to treat acute Q fever. Chronic Q fever requires prolonged treatment with antibiotics.

## THE Q FEVER VACCINE

An inactivated vaccine (Q-Vax®), given under the skin, has been available in Australia since 1989. A clinical trial involving 200 abattoir workers who received the vaccine reported that after 15 months of follow-up, there were seven cases of Q fever in the control group and no cases in the vaccinated group (Shapiro, 1990). Complete immunity was achieved after 10 to 15 days, and immunity tends to persist. Vaccination has reduced the incidence of Q fever in Australia (Marmion, 2007). This vaccine is not available in the UK or the U.S. Vaccination is recommended for people aged 15 years or older at risk of infection with *C. burnetii* (ATAGI, 2025d). However, the vaccine can induce local reactions, and patients should be evaluated with a skin test before vaccination. This initial test is given to avoid severe side-effects, such as an abscess at the injection site, muscle pain, fever and headaches. You should also have a blood test to check for pre-existing immunity.

About 10% of Q-Vax recipients experience mild influenza-like symptoms, such as headache, fever, chills or minor sweating.

**If you're about to start cancer treatment and you work with animals or in rural areas, ask your doctor whether a Q fever skin test and vaccine is appropriate for you.**

## SHOULD I BE VACCINATED FOR Q FEVER?

Patients with who have an unexplained fever and who live in areas in which *C. burnetii* is common should undergo blood testing to detect this microorganism (Raoult, 1992).

Immunosuppressed patients are said to be more prone to developing chronic Q fever. If you're at risk of Q fever, I suggest that you have the vaccine before starting your cancer treatment. Although Q-Vax is inactivated, it is not recommended during cancer treatment or while your immune system is suppressed. This is because there isn't enough evidence that the vaccine is safe or effective when your immune defences are low (ATAGI, 2025d; TGA, 2019).

## THE Q FEVER REGISTER

In 2002, a national register was established by the Australian meat and livestock industry to assist workers and employers monitor their immunity to Q fever. In April 2024, the Australian Q Fever Register merged with the Australian Immunisation Register (AIR), so all information regarding Q fever vaccination and immunity should now be reported to the AIR.

**For more information, see https://www.health.gov.au/news/addition-of-q-fever-vaccines-to-the-australian-immunisation-register.**

# 9

# OTHER VACCINES

## HEPATITIS B VACCINE

Hepatitis B virus (HBV) may be reactivated if you have chemotherapy. Therefore, HBV status is usually checked before you start chemotherapy. Susceptible higher-risk groups (including healthcare workers, sex workers, and drug users) should be immunised at the time of diagnosis. Patients at higher risk, such as those who have undergone a bone marrow transplant, should also have three doses of hepatitis B vaccine administered six to 12 months after their transplant (**Table 10.1**).

## HUMAN PAPILLOMA VIRUS (HPV) VACCINE

HPV is associated with various illnesses, including genital warts and cancer of the cervix, vulva, vagina, penis or anus. There is an increased incidence of HPV-related cancers for HIV/AIDS patients or after a bone marrow transplant (Grulich, 2007). The ACIP and the CDC advise routine vaccination for males and females aged 11 to 12 years old. For those not vaccinated, catch-up vaccination is recommended for people up to 26 years old.

In 2019, the CDC announced that catch-up vaccinations could be given to all adults aged 27 to 45, regardless of sex, based on shared clinical decision-making (Meites, 2019). This recommendation remains in place as of 2025.

The NCCN Guidelines® for Prevention and Treatment of Cancer-Related Infections recommend the HPV vaccine for previously unvaccinated cancer survivors up to 45 years of age (NCCN, 2025).

The Australian Immunisation Handbook advises that a three-dose schedule of 9vHPV vaccine is recommended for people with significant immunocompromising conditions, regardless of their age when they started vaccination (ATAGI, 2025b).

Significant immunocompromising conditions include:

- primary or secondary immunodeficiencies (complete or partial deficiencies of B-lymphocyte antibody or T-lymphocytes)
- HIV infection
- malignancy
- organ transplantation
- significant immunosuppressive therapy.

## MEASLES-MUMPS-RUBELLA (MMR) VACCINE

The MMR vaccine is a live vaccine containing attenuated (weakened) viruses, and great care needs to be taken if you have had cancer treatment and may have ongoing immunosuppression. This vaccine should not be given during periods of significant immunosuppression. Adults who do not have evidence of immunity should get at least one dose of MMR vaccine. Evidence means that you have documented proof of vaccination or previous disease diagnosed by a doctor, or you have laboratory evidence of immunity (i.e., results of a blood test).

Some adults may need two doses of MMR. Adults who will be in a setting that poses a high risk for measles or mumps transmission should make sure they have had two doses separated by at least 28 days. These adults include:

- students at post-high school education institutions
- healthcare personnel
- international travellers.

For cancer patients, MMR should only be considered if your immunity is not suppressed three or more months after chemotherapy, six months or longer after anti-B antibody therapy (such as rituximab), and 24 months after a bone marrow transplant. Consultation with an infectious disease clinician is strongly advised.

## MENINGOCOCCAL VACCINE

*Neisseria meningitidis* causes meningococcal disease and is also known as meningococcus. There are 13 known meningococcal serogroups. Invasive meningococcal disease (IMD) is a rare but serious disease that can present as septicaemia, with or without meningitis. Vaccination is routine in children and young adults and may be advised if you have had a bone marrow transplant. Consult your haematologist or infectious diseases specialist if:

- you are considered high-risk
- you work in a laboratory handling *N. meningitidis*
- there is a local outbreak
- you have had your spleen removed.

## HAEMOPHILUS INFLUENZAE TYPE B (HIB) VACCINE

*Haemophilus influenzae* is a bug that is a normal part of the upper airways of the throat and lung. Hib can cause serious diseases in children and in people who are immunocompromised, including bacterial meningitis, pneumonia, epiglottitis, septic arthritis and cellulitis.

Hib-containing vaccine is recommended routinely for infants and children and people who are immunocompromised, such as those who have had a bone marrow transplant (**Table 10.1**).

## RESPIRATORY SYNCYTIAL VIRUS (RSV) VACCINE

RSV is a common virus that can cause serious illness, especially in older adults, babies, and people with weakened immune systems. It can lead to lung infections like pneumonia and bronchiolitis. Bronchiolitis is an infection that causes the small airways in the lungs to become swollen and blocked, making it hard to breathe. RSV can also make existing breathing problems worse, such as asthma or smoking-related lung disease; in some cases it can cause people to be hospitalised with breathing diliculties or even die.

In 2023, two vaccines – Arexvy® by GSK, and Abrysvo® by Pfizer – were approved for use in adults aged 60 years and older. In Australia, these vaccines are available on private prescription but are not yet part of the NIP for older adults. Abrysvo is also funded for pregnant women between 28 and 36 weeks' gestation to help protect newborns in their first few months of life.

A recent study showed that many people with weakened immune systems, including cancer survivors, still respond well to the Arexvy vaccine and may gain protection from serious illness (Karaba, 2025). If you are over 60 and have had chemotherapy or a bone marrow transplant, ask your doctor whether RSV vaccination is right for you.

There is a small risk of Guillain-Barré syndrome (GBS), a rare nerve condition, after RSV vaccination. This occurred in a few people in a large U.S. study. The estimated risk of GBS is about 1 in 200,000 for Arexvy and 1 in 55,000 for Abrysvo (Fry, 2025). While this risk is low, it's worth discussing the pros and cons with your doctor.

## YELLOW FEVER VACCINE

Yellow fever is a serious mosquito-borne viral infection found in parts of Africa and South America. Some countries require proof of vaccination for entry. The yellow fever vaccine is a live vaccine, given by injection, and is highly effective – one dose typically provides lifelong protection. However, because it is a live vaccine, it is not recommended for people with weakened immune systems, including those undergoing or recovering from cancer treatment, or people who have had a bone marrow transplant. If you are unable to receive the vaccine, your doctor may provide a medical exemption certificate. The vaccine should be given at least 10 days before travel to allow time for immunity to develop. Mild side-effects such as headache or fever are common; serious reactions are rare. The yellow fever vaccine is available only at approved travel vaccination centres and is documented on an international certificate of vaccination, which may be required at international borders.

## TRAVEL VACCINATION

Before travelling, consider referral to a travel medicine specialist. If you have just completed chemotherapy or are immunosuppressed, avoid live vaccines, including oral polio and oral typhoid vaccines. Hepatitis A, injectable polio and injectable typhoid vaccines are considered safe. If possible, defer travel and avoid high-risk countries with limited health infrastructure.

**If you are planning overseas travel within six months of cancer treatment, speak to a travel medicine specialist to tailor your vaccination schedule.**

# 10

# VACCINES AFTER A BONE MARROW TRANSPLANT

## TYPES OF BONE MARROW TRANSPLANTS

A bone marrow transplant, also known as a stem cell transplant, is a procedure used to restore stem cells after cancer treatment. Some people with cancer (particularly blood cancers) are given high doses of chemotherapy, sometimes combined with radiation therapy, to kill the cancer cells in their body. However, this treatment also kills healthy stem cells in the bone marrow that produce your blood. A bone marrow transplant involves transfusing healthy stem cells into the body so they can produce new red blood cells, white blood cells, and platelets.

Bone marrow transplants are categorised as 'autologous', when your own bone marrow is used, or 'allogeneic', when another person's bone marrow is used. The transplanted marrow and/or stem cells make their way via the bloodstream into your bone marrow and start to produce new blood cells. You will then need to be re-vaccinated when your immune system has at least partially recovered.

Graft-versus-host disease (GVHD) occurs when types of white blood cells (T cells) in the donated bone marrow (i.e., from an allogeneic transplant) attack your body's cells that they see as foreign.

## AM I AT HIGHER RISK OF COVID-19 OR OTHER INFECTIONS AFTER A TRANSPLANT?

Patients with cancer affecting the bone marrow or lymphatic system and recipients of bone marrow transplants have severely depressed immunity. You will be more prone to infection due to prior intensive therapies and the drugs used to prevent and treat GVHD. Antibody levels in your blood against pneumonia and influenza drop significantly and you must start your vaccinations all over again.

Varicella (chickenpox) in patients who have lost their pre-existing immunity **(seronegative)**, or shingles in **seropositive** patients, can be serious after a bone marrow transplant. Long-term antiviral drugs such as aciclovir are usually required.

In addition, you are at a high risk of complications and death from COVID-19, comparable to the mortality rate of aged-care residents. The risk is exceptionally high for patients over the age of 60 or those who are hospitalised (Vijenthira, 2020).

Household transmission is one of the most common mechanisms of COVID-19 transmission. As a result, COVID-19 vaccination of this group of patients, their carers and their families is a priority, as indicated in a statement from the Australia and New Zealand Transplant and Cellular Therapies group (ANZTCT, 2021).

If you've had an autologous transplant (using your own stem cells), you should be able to have the COVID-19 vaccine two months after the transplant. If you've had an allogeneic transplant (using donor stem cells), you should be able to have the vaccine from three to six months after the transplant. These recommendations can change over time, so keep in touch with your treatment team and refer to trusted websites from official health organisations for current guidelines.

In August 2021, the FDA approved a third dose of the Pfizer or Moderna vaccine for people with significantly weakened immune systems, including those who had received an organ transplant. Since then, guidelines have evolved to include patients who have received a bone marrow or stem cell transplant. A third dose is now considered part of the COVID-19 primary vaccine course for these individuals, ideally given at least 28 days after the second dose of the vaccine and at least three months after transplant, depending on your immune recovery. If you've had a stem cell transplant or are on ongoing immunosuppressive therapy, discuss the timing and type of vaccines with your treating team. The first and second doses of the primary course are usually spaced three to eight weeks apart, depending on the particular vaccine and clinical situation.

In both Australia and the UK, national immunisation guidelines also recommend a third primary dose of COVID-19 vaccine for severely immunocompromised individuals, including post-transplant patients, followed by booster doses depending on your age and risk level.

## WHEN CAN I HAVE MY ROUTINE VACCINATIONS?

**Table 10.1** summarises the Australian guidelines for revaccination following a bone marrow transplant. (ATAGI uses the term HSCT, which stands for haematopoietic stem cell transplant/transplantation.) Vaccination schedules may differ depending on available vaccine brands, timing of immune recovery, and local public health policies.

| Vaccine | Start (time after HSCT) | Dosing schedule |
|---|---|---|
| BCG | | |
| COVID-19 | 3–6 months | 2–3 primary doses, then booster doses every 6–12 months as needed |
| Hib | 6 months | 3 doses |
| Hepatitis B | 6 months | 3 doses |
| Human papilloma virus | 6 months, but immune response may be enhanced by waiting until 12 months | 3 doses |
| Influenza | 3–6 months | 2 doses in the first year, then annually |
| Measles, mumps, rubella (MMR) | 24 months; consider a blood test to confirm need for revaccination. | 2 doses |
| Meningococcal disease | 6 months | • MenACWY vaccine: 2 primary doses + booster every 5 years<br>• MenB vaccine: 2 primary doses + a single booster 5 years later |
| Pneumococcal disease | 3–6 months | 3 doses of PCV followed by 1 dose of PPSV23, then a booster of PPSV23 ≥5 years later |
| Polio | 6 months | 3 doses |
| RSV | 3–6 months | Adults ≥60: 1 dose |
| Shingles (zoster) | 6 months, in adults >18 | 2 doses |
| Tetanus, diphtheria, pertussis | 6 months | 3 doses |
| Varicella | 24 months | 2 doses |

**Table 10.1**

Recommended vaccination schedule for adults in Australia following stem cell or bone marrow transplant (ATAGI, 2025e).

| Minimum dose interval | Comments |
| --- | --- |
| | Not recommended after HSCT. |
| 4 weeks | Consider a third primary dose. Additional doses based on age and other individual risk factors. |
| 4 weeks | |
| 1–2 months between dose 1 & 2, and 3 months between dose 2 & 3 | High-dose formulation (H-B-Vax II dialysis formulation) is preferred. If not available, give single-strength hepatitis B vaccine in each arm at each dosing interval. |
| 1–2 months between dose 1 & 2, and 4 months between dose 2 & 3 | For adults >25, give on a case-by-case basis, depending on risk. |
| 4 weeks | May start earlier if outbreak; annual flu vaccine in following years, usually in autumn. |
| 4 weeks | Live vaccine; consider if no immunosuppression or GVHD. Check serology 4–6 weeks after the first dose. |
| • MenACWY: 8 weeks<br>• MenB: 4 weeks | 2 vaccines available to cover different serogroups. Dose, brand and timing vary by age; shown here is the advice for adults. |
| 2 months | If a person receives 21vPCV as their PCV dose, the subsequent doses of PPSV23 are not required. |
| 4 weeks | A 10-yearly booster dose is recommended for people with ongoing polio exposure. |
| | |
| 4 weeks | Use Shingrix. Consider delaying the timing of each dose (e.g., dose 1 at 7 months and dose 2 at 9 months) as needed. |
| 4 weeks | Use dTpa vaccine for people ≥10 years old. |
| 4 weeks | Live vaccine; consider if no immunosuppression or GVHD. |

Note: Live vaccines usually considered ≥ 24 months post-HSCT if immune recovery confirmed. Advice not applicable to adults has been omitted; refer to Aust. Immunisation Handbook for complete table.

The advice in **Table 10.1** comes from the Australian Immunisation Handbook. For international recommendations, consult the sections related to immunosuppressed or at-risk populations in the vaccination guidelines of other countries. For example, see 'immunisation of immunocompromised persons' in the Canadian Immunization Guide (Public Health Agency of Canada, 2024); the CDC guidelines for 'altered immunocompetence' (CDC, 2024a), or the UK government's Green Book, particularly chapters 6 and 7 (UKHSA, 2025).

For information specific to HSCT, you can also look to guidelines and consensus statements published by professional societies such as the Infectious Diseases Society of America (Rubin, 2014), the British Society of Blood and Marrow Transplantation and Cellular Therapy (Miller, 2023), or the European Group of Blood and Marrow Transplantation (EBMT). The EBMT Handbook has a whole chapter about vaccinations for transplant recipients (de la Cámara, 2024).

Always consult your transplant team or infectious diseases specialist, as their advice for you may vary depending on the type of transplant you received and how long ago you had it, your GVHD status, and how well your immune system has recovered. (See also Kamboj, 2019; Cordonnier, 2019.)

The information provided in this chapter may not necessarily apply to your situation. Book in a longer consultation with your doctor, haematology nurse or pharmacist to work through these questions. Remember, one size doesn't fit all; although the guidelines appear prescriptive and may say you should wait for six months after your transplant, it often doesn't really matter if the timing is four, six, eight or 12 months later for many vaccines. You may have so much going on with getting back to your life and work, or just managing the ups and downs of your recovery, that a few weeks here or there won't make an enormous difference.

One important message consistent in all the guidelines is that high-risk patients should not receive live vaccines (such as MMR or varicella/zoster) until at least two years have elapsed after transplant, there is no evidence of GVHD, and all medications that reduce immunity have been ceased. Carpenter (2016) advised the '2-1-8 rule': no live vaccines until you are at least two years out from bone marrow transplant, one year off immunosuppressive therapy and eight months from any prior doses of intravenous immunoglobulin (IVIG).

## SHOULD I DELAY MY VACCINATION IF I HAVE GRAFT-VERSUS-HOST DISEASE?

GVHD is relatively common after an allogeneic transplant and can either be short-lived or become a chronic problem. GVHD can cause a range of symptoms, such as a skin rash or liver and abdominal symptoms. It can be serious, and the drugs used to treat it will suppress your immune system.

An excellent review from the University of Washington advises patients with moderate or severe GVHD to reconsider vaccinations 12 months after transplantation. The reason for this delay is that your immune system will still be suppressed, and you may not achieve a sufficient immune response from the vaccine. For patients with late-onset chronic GVHD, blood tests are recommended to measure the immune cells in the blood. If the CD4 level is greater than 200 and CD19 is 20 or more, you will be considered eligible to start conjugated vaccines such as those to protect against *H. influenzae*, pneumococcal disease and meningitis (Carpenter, 2016).

Even once you've had the COVID-19 vaccine, it is still essential to take precautions against infection, as we don't yet know how much protection the vaccine provides for people who've had a stem cell transplant. A review of studies on COVID-19 vaccination in different immunocompromised populations found that there was limited information about how well it works in stem cell recipients (Galmiche, 2022).

One small study from Israel, in which 66 patients received the Pfizer COVID-19 vaccine after an allogeneic bone marrow transplant, is reassuring in its results. In this study, a minimum of three months between the transplant and vaccination was required. Overall, the vaccine was well tolerated. Twelve per cent of the patients experienced a drop in blood count after the first dose, and 10% after the second dose, and there were three cases of GVHD becoming worse. A single case of impending graft rejection was summarised as possibly related. However, the immune response to the vaccine was a high 75% (Ram, 2021).

## WHAT IF I AM HAVING THERAPY THAT REDUCES MY B-CELL COUNT?

If you are receiving anti-CD20 monoclonal antibodies, such as rituximab, obinutuzumab or other B-cell depleting therapies, you may not have an adequate antibody response to vaccines.

Drugs specifically targeted against B-cells (e.g., venetoclax, ibrutinib and acalabrutinib) are increasingly being used for diseases such as chronic lymphatic leukaemia, mantle cell lymphoma and Waldenstrom macroglobulinemia, and may also impair your response to vaccination. Ibrutinib has also been used for patients with GVHD when other treatments have failed. If you are on these types of therapies, it would be best to wait for at least six months after your last dose before getting vaccinated. In one study of influenza vaccination for patients on rituximab, there was a recovery of vaccine responsiveness to 50% at six months and to normal responsiveness 12 months after exposure (de Lavallade, 2011).

These types of therapies can make vaccination advice challenging. For example, studies of influenza vaccine with ibrutinib have shown inconsistent results, with one study showing an impaired response (Douglas, 2017) and another study showing a good response in at least 25% of recipients, possibly due to the stronger adjuvanted vaccine used for some of their patients (Sun, 2016). Always consult your haematologist about the optimal timing of vaccines for you.

Antibody levels after COVID-19 vaccination are lower than the lowest levels of a normal population by 33% for patients with haematological malignancy, 17% for those who have had a bone marrow transplant and 10% for people with solid cancers. For patients with vasculitis on rituximab, the antibody response was reduced by 87% (Kearns, 2021). On a more positive note, a another study showed that 75% of patients given Shingrix while on drugs targeting their B cells developed a strong immune response to the vaccine (Zent, 2021).

## VACCINATION AFTER CHIMERIC ANTIGEN RECEPTOR (CAR) T-CELL THERAPY

In 2017, the first CAR T-cell therapies were approved by the FDA for the treatment of refractory acute lymphoblastic leukaemia (ALL) in children and young adults, and advanced B-cell lymphomas in adult patients.

In recent years, CAR T-cell therapies have also been approved for the treatment of mantle cell lymphoma and multiple myeloma. Using genetic engineering technology, these T cells learn to recognise and destroy specific antigens on tumour cells. CAR T cells destroy not only specific tumour cells but also healthy B and T cells, which weakens your immune system and leaves you vulnerable to infections (Riedel, 2025).

If you've had CAR T-cell therapy, you are classified as being severely immunocompromised for the first 24 months. During this period, live vaccines are not recommended; while it's safe to receive other vaccines, they may work less well and require extra doses (ATAGI, 2025f). Discuss this with your treatment team.

There is some emerging data from Israel that close to 60% of patients with a prior CAR T infusion had evidence of COVID-19 immunity after the Pfizer vaccine (Ram, 2021).

# 11

# PREPARING FOR VACCINATION

## HOW DO I PREPARE FOR MY VACCINATION APPOINTMENT?



The following lists offer some key points to think about before you are vaccinated. The exact process will vary depending on the region where you live. When I took my mother to be vaccinated for COVID-19, she was scared and anxious. The media hype in Australia about potential side-effects didn't help the situation. Talk to your family or support person about your fears.

- Attend your vaccination appointment with a family member, carer, or friend, particularly if you are elderly.
- Get to your appointment early as there may be consent forms to complete.
- Bring country-specific health IDs such as your Medicare or other health cards.
- Bring a face mask in case you are required to wear one at your appointment.
- Wear loose clothing that allows easy access to your upper arm, where you will receive the vaccine.
- Bring a book or phone/tablet to keep you busy while waiting.
- Continue your usual medications, including vitamins and any anti-cancer treatments, unless advised otherwise by your doctor.
- If you are attending your regular medical clinic, they will know you well and have a copy of your medical record.
- If you are attending a vaccination centre, take a letter from your general practitioner or make a summary of your medications and prior health conditions. Take a printed copy of your medical record if possible. Importantly, make a list of your allergies and any reactions you've had. For example, did you have an allergic reaction to chemotherapy or other medication, and if so, was it mild or severe?
- If you have had severe allergies, see your immunologist, and attend a vaccination a centre where there is plenty of on-site medical support on-site, including doctors.

## WHAT HAPPENS WHEN I AM BEING VACCINATED?

- You will be asked to go to a vaccination bay or room, where the person vaccinating you will:
  - take your consent form, if any
  - confirm your identity
  - ask about your recent vaccination history
  - ask about past allergies
  - obtain your informed consent for the delivery of the vaccine and check your signature
  - administer your vaccine.
- The vaccine will be administered into the muscle of your upper arm by a nurse, pharmacist, doctor, or other healthcare worker.
- If you have had cancer surgery to your arm or armpit, you can request that they use the other side, given the rare possibility of lymphoedema after your injection.
- If you're taking any blood-thinners, let the vaccinator know beforehand and apply pressure over the injection site afterwards for at least five minutes.

## WHAT HAPPENS AFTER MY VACCINATION?

- After you have been vaccinated, you will leave your consent form with the vaccinator and they will provide you with a vaccine record.
- You will typically be observed for at least 15 minutes after being vaccinated to ensure you don't experience any immediate reactions.
- If you have a history of allergic reactions (including food allergies, reactions to insect stings or medicine allergies), you will be observed for 30 minutes.
- If you are elderly and live alone, consider asking somebody to stay with you for the night or stay in close contact with them by phone.
- If you experience any unusual or severe side-effects, call your doctor or an ambulance.

- Your upper arm and lymph nodes under your armpit may become sore, so don't hesitate to take some Panadol/Tylenol if it starts to ache or becomes sore. You may find it hard to sleep on that side for a few days after the injection.

## CONCLUSION AND SUMMARY

I'm sorry to admit that advice regarding vaccination after cancer treatment is often fragmented within the medical profession. There is a lot of information that I've included in this book, and I do not expect you to remember it all. Instead, I have summarised some key information in the following tables. **Table 11.1** lists important vaccines for cancer patients with the recommended timings to fit around your cancer treatment. The final table (**Table 11.2**) summarises all the vaccines mentioned throughout the book, with some brief recommendations and chapter links for further reading. This table is based on information from the Australian Immunisation Handbook as well as the American Society of Clinical Oncology (ASCO) guidelines (Kamboj, 2024).

Vaccination is important, and I urge you to take control of this aspect of your survivorship journey. This book is intended to be a helpful guide, but continue to check online sources such as the Australian Immunisation Handbook, CDC website and other health organisations for up-to-date information. Websites and articles that we have cited can also be used for further reading. Discuss any issues with your treating team, including your general practitioner, oncologist or haematologist. Taking control will help you protect yourself against preventable diseases. Best wishes and God bless.

| Vaccine | Before chemotherapy | During chemotherapy | After chemotherapy |
|---|---|---|---|
| COVID-19 | Yes, >2 weeks before starting chemo | Between cycles, e.g., Days 1–3 or Day 21 of chemo given every 3 weeks, avoiding the period of lowest white cell count (the **nadir**), or if you have a fever. | Yes. Wait at least 1 month, or give immediately if high prevalence of COVID-19. |
| Influenza | Yes, >2 weeks before starting chemo | Between cycles (as above) | Yes. Wait at least 1 month. |
| Pneumococcal disease | Yes – if you are starting chemo within 3 months, have a single dose of PCV13 (to be followed by PPSV23 after chemo is completed) | No | Yes, at least 2 months after chemo.<br>Wait longer if you had more intensive treatment (e.g., 6 months for leukaemia patients) |
| Shingles (zoster) | Yes, 1–4 weeks before chemo | Yes | Yes, at least 2 months after chemo. |
| Tetanus, diptheria, pertussis | Yes, if previously unvaccinated or >10 years since your last dose | No | Wait at least 3 months. |

**Table 11.1**
Vaccination for people with cancer: recommended timing in relation to treatment.

| During radiation therapy | During hormonal therapy | Comments |
|---|---|---|
| Yes | Yes | **Strongly advised**<br>Ensure regular boosters every 6–12 months, depending on your individual level of risk. Avoid injection on the same side as previous breast or arm surgery. Can be given with the flu shot. |
| Yes | Yes | **Advised yearly**<br>• Not nasal spray (live flu vaccine)<br>• Take care with immunotherapy such as pembrolizumab |
| Yes | Yes | **Strongly advised**<br>In Australia/UK, PCV13 is followed by 1 dose of PPSV23 8–52 weeks after finishing chemo, plus a booster dose 5 years later.<br>In the USA, PCV20 or PCV21 is preferred as a one-off pre-treatment vaccine; if PCV15 is used, follow with PPSV23 at least 8 weeks after chemo. |
| Yes | | **Strongly advised**<br>If you were previously vaccinated with Zostavax (discontinued), you can still receive Shingrix, though it may not be funded. |
| If clinically indicated (e.g., new wound or injury) | Yes | **Advised**<br>If you're an adult and were never vaccinated, or if you are severely immunosuppressed, you may need more than one dose. |

Note: Funding is not available in all circumstances. Guidelines can change over time, as new information becomes available or new vaccines are developed. Always check with your healthcare provider and refer to up-to-date, country-specific guidelines.

| Vaccine-preventable disease | Vaccine type | Recom-mended | Optional (special conditions) |
|---|---|---|---|
| Cholera | | | ✓ |
| COVID-19 | mRNA, protein subunit | ✓ | |
| Diphtheria | dTpa, dT | ✓ | |
| *H. influenzae* type B | Hib | | ✓ |
| Hepatitis A | HepA, HepA-HepB | | ✓ |
| Hepatitis B | HepB, HepA-HepB | ✓ | |
| Human papilloma virus | 9vHPV | ✓ | |
| Influenza | trivalent, quadrivalent | ✓ | |
| Japanese encephalitis | | | ✓ |
| Measles, mumps, rubella | MMR | ✓ | |
| Meningococcal disease | MenACWY, MenB | | ✓ |
| Pertussis (whooping cough) | dTpa | ✓ | |
| Pneumococcal disease | PPSV, PCV | ✓ | |
| Polio | IPV, dTpa-IPV | | ✓ |
| Q fever | Q-Vax | | ✓ |
| RSV | recombinant (e.g. Arexvy) | ✓ | |
| Tetanus | dTpa, dT | ✓ | |
| Tuberculosis | BCG | | ✓ |
| Typhoid | ViCPS | | ✓ |
| Varicella | monovalent (e.g. Varivax) | | ✓ |
| Yellow fever | | | ✓ |
| Zoster (shingles) | RZV (Shingrix) | ✓ | |

**Table 11.2**
Summary of vaccine recommendations for adults with cancer.

| Caution: live vaccine? | Comments, recommendations, special conditions | Chapter |
|---|---|---|
| | Travel vaccine; use inactivated form (Dukoral). | |
| | Continue every 6–12 months. | 4 |
| | Booster every 10 years. | |
| | Recommended after HSCT (see Table 10.1). | 9 |
| | Travel, occupational exposure (lab/sewage work), chronic liver disease, HIV, lifestyle risk factors e.g. drug use, higher-risk sexual exposure | 9 |
| | Travel, receiving blood products, occupational exposure, drug use, HIV. | 9 |
| | Age 19–26, vaccinate; 27–45, shared decision-making (U.S.). No age limit in Australia. | 9 |
| | Continue every year. Use injectable form (no live nasal spray). | 3 |
| | Travel vaccine; use inactivated form (JEspect). | |
| | Live vaccines not safe if immunocompromised. MMRV not suitable for adults. | 9 |
| | Recommended after HSCT (see Table 10.1). | 9 |
| | Booster every 10 years. | 7 |
| | Dosing schedule depends on type of vaccine available. | 6 |
| | Travel, childhood catch-up, or after HSCT (see Table 10.1). Use injectable form. | 9 |
| N | Occupational exposure (working with animals). Avoid if immunocompromised. | 8 |
| | Single dose for adults ≥60, or ≥50 with medical condtions. | 9 |
| | Booster every 10 years. | |
| | Occupational exposure (healthcare workers) or high-risk travel. Not usually recommended for cancer patients; seek specialist advice. | |
| | Travel vaccine; use injectable form. | 9 |
| | If no evidence of immunity. MMRV not suitable for adults. | 10 |
| Y | Occupational exposure (lab workers) or high-risk travel. | 9 |
| | For immunocompromised adults ≥18 and healthy adults ≥50. | 5 |

# Endnotes

## CREDITS

**Editing and proofreading:** Felicity Sutton

**Cover and book design:** John Bull, Publishing Art Australia

Photo of John being vaccinated ©BC Publishing Pty Ltd

**Figure 1.1:** ©BC Publishing Pty Ltd

**Figure 2.1:** iStock Images, under licence (fstop123)

**Figure 3.1:** Shutterstock Images, under licence (Drazen Zigic)

**Figure 5.1:** Shutterstock Images, under licence (MR.samoraphum suksamran)

## DISCLAIMERS

Reference to specific commercial products, manufacturers, companies, or trademarks does not constitute its endorsement or recommendation by the U.S. Government, Department of Health and Human Services, or Centers for Disease Control and Prevention.

NCCN makes no warranties of any kind whatsoever regarding their content, use or application and disclaims any responsibility for their application or use in any way.

Information referenced from the NCCN Clinical Practice Guidelines in Oncology (NCCN Guidelines®) for Prevention and Treatment of Cancer-Related Infections V.1.2025. © National Comprehensive Cancer Network, Inc. 2025. All rights reserved. Accessed September 2, 2025. To view the most recent and complete version of the guideline, go online to NCCN.org.

## ABBREVIATIONS

**ACIP:** Advisory Committee on Immunization Practices [USA]

**ATAGI:** Australian Technical Advisory Group on Immunisation

**CAR:** chimeric antigen receptor

**CDC:** U.S. Centers for Disease Control and Prevention

**DTPa/DTaP or dTpa/Tdap:** diphtheria, tetanus, and acellular pertussis-containing vaccine

**EBMT:** European Group of Blood and Marrow Transplantation

**FDA:** U.S. Food and Drug Administration

**GBS:** Guillain-Barré syndrome

**GVHD:** graft-versus-host disease

**HBV:** hepatitis B virus

**HIV:** human immunodeficiency virus

**ICIs:** immune checkpoint inhibitors

**IPD:** invasive pneumococcal disease

**JCVI:** Joint Committee on Vaccination and Immunisation [UK]

**MMR:** measles, mumps, rubella (combination vaccine)

**mRNA:** messenger ribonucleic acid

**NIP:** National Immunisation Program [Australia]

**NCCN:** National Comprehensive Cancer Network [USA]

**PCV:** pneumococcal conjugate vaccine

**PPSV:** pneumococcal polysaccharide vaccine

**TTS:** thrombosis with thrombocytopenia syndrome

## GLOSSARY

**adjuvanted:** containing a substance (adjuvant) which has been added to increase the immune response, e.g., to create a 'stronger' vaccine

**anaphylaxis:** a sudden and severe allergic reaction to an antigen (e.g., a bee sting) to which the body has become oversensitive

**antibody:** a blood protein produced in response to a specific antigen

**antigen:** a foreign substance such as a germ that induces an immune response in the body, especially the production of antibodies

**attenuated vaccine:** a weakened form of the germ (antigen) which normally makes you sick that induces antibodies to produce immunity

**bacteria:** microorganisms that are smaller than a blood cell but larger than a virus and usually respond to antibiotics

**booster:** an extra dose of a vaccine given to maintain protection against a disease. Many vaccines induce immunity that wear off over time, requiring additional doses.

**checkpoint protein:** a protein produced by cancer cells to help them evade the body's immune system

**combined vaccine:** two or more vaccines given in a single dose to protect against more than one disease

**conjugate vaccine:** a vaccine containing a polysaccharide antigen joined (conjugated) to a carrier molecule, which enhances the stability and the effectiveness of the vaccine

**contagious:** able to be transmitted from one person to another through casual touch, sexual activity, or body fluids

**COVID-19:** an infectious disease caused by the SARS-CoV-2 virus, discovered in 2019. 'CO' stands for corona, 'VI' for virus, and 'D' for disease.

**dermatome:** a band or region of skin supplied by a single nerve responsible for sensation

**graft-versus-host disease (GVHD):** a condition that occurs when donated stem cells or bone marrow attack the recipient's body after a transplant. This is because T cells in the transplant (graft) see the other cells in the body (host) as foreign.

**Guillain–Barré syndrome:** an autoimmune condition that causes muscle weakness, numbness, or paralysis

**haematological malignancy:** cancer that develops in the blood cells, including leukaemia, lymphoma and myeloma

**haematoma:** a solid swelling of clotted blood within the tissues, usually associated with a bruise

**immune response:** the reaction of the body's immune system to the presence of a foreign substance (antigen)

**immune system:** the organs and processes in the body that provide resistance to viruses, bacteria and other toxins. Organs include the thymus, spleen, bone marrow and lymph nodes.

**immunisation:** the process of inducing immunity to a virus, toxoid, or bacteria by giving a vaccine

**immunocompromised:** having a weakened immune system.

**immunosuppression:** the partial or complete suppression of the immune response of an individual, e.g., with steroid medication

**inactivated vaccine:** a vaccine containing a pathogen that has been killed or made ineffective, so is unable to replicate inside the body or cause disease, but which still triggers the immune system

**intradermal injection:** an injection into the dermis of the skin, which lies just below the skin surface

**intramuscular injection:** an injection into the muscle. Vaccines are usually injected into a muscle in the upper arm or upper outer thigh.

**live vaccine:** any preparation of weakened (attenuated) or killed bacteria or virus, introduced into the body to prevent disease by stimulating antibodies against it

**lymphadenitis:** inflammation of the lymph nodes, usually in the armpit as a reaction to an infection or vaccination in the arm

**lymphocytes:** a type of white blood cell; the two main types are B lymphocytes (B cells), which make antibodies, and T lymphocytes (T cells), which help kill foreign bodies.

**lymphoedema:** localised swelling of the body caused by an abnormal accumulation of lymphatic fluid

**meta-analysis:** examination of large amounts of data from numerous independent studies of the same subject to determine overall trends

**monovalent:** active against a single antigen, microorganism, or disease

**mRNA vaccine:** a new type of vaccine to protect against infectious diseases. They teach our cells how to make a protein, or just a piece of a protein, which triggers an immune response inside our bodies.

**nadir:** the period in a chemotherapy cycle in which your blood counts are at their lowest (often about 10–14 days after treatment)

**pandemic:** an outbreak of a disease that occurs over a wide geographic area and infects a large proportion of individuals

**placebo:** a substance or treatment designed to have no therapeutic value that is given in the same way as a treatment being tested

**platelet:** a type of blood cell involved in clotting

**polysaccharide vaccine:** a type of vaccine that contains a group of complex carbohydrates (sugars) that make up the cell coating of the bacterium

**polyvalent:** active against several toxins or strains of a pathogen

**postherpetic neuralgia:** a condition of recurring or persistent pain and abnormal burning sensation in an area of the body which has undergone an outbreak of shingles

**prophylaxis:** treatment given, or action taken, to prevent disease

**seronegative:** containing no detectable antibodies in the blood for a particular disease or vaccine

**seropositive:** having detectable antibodies against a specific antigen in the blood

**shingles (zoster):** a painful skin eruption, often forming a band around the middle of the body, caused by the same virus that causes chickenpox

**solid malignancy:** cancer that develops in body organs or tissues (e.g., breast, prostate, lung), forming a solid tumour.

**T cell:** a type of white blood cell that helps protect the body by identifying and attacking foreign cells including viruses, toxins and cancer

**thrombocytopenia:** deficiency of platelets in the blood, which can cause bleeding into the tissues, bruising and slow blood-clotting

**thrombosis:** formation of blood clots in veins or arteries

**toxoplasmosis:** a disease transmitted in uncooked meats, soil and cat faeces

**virus:** a tiny, living organism that can replicate itself and cause disease

## REFERENCES

**American Society for Radiation Oncology (ASTRO).** Ask a radiation oncologist: radiation therapy for breast cancer. ASTRO (2021): https://www.rtanswers.org/RTAnswers/media/RTAnswers/Ask%20a%20Radiation%20Oncologist/PDFs/AaRO_BreastSlides.pdf

**Australia and New Zealand Transplant and Cellular Therapies Limited (ANZTCT).** COVID-19 vaccination consensus position statement 20th January 2021. ANZTCT (2021): https://anztct.org.au/anztct-covid-19-vaccination-position-statement/

**Australian Institute of Health and Welfare (AIHW).** Fact sheet: shingles in Australia. AIHW (2025), available at: https://www.aihw.gov.au/reports/immunisation/vaccine-preventable-diseases/contents/fact-sheets

**Australian Technical Advisory Group on Immunisation (ATAGI).** ATAGI statement on the administration of COVID-19 vaccines in 2024. Department of Health, Disability and Ageing (2024a): https://www.health.gov.au/resources/publications/atagi-statement-on-the-administration-of-covid-19-vaccines-in-2024

**ATAGI.** Risk conditions and immunosuppressive therapies for zoster vaccination and eligibility for NIP funding. Australian Immunisation Handbook, Department of Health, Disability and Ageing (2024b): https://immunisationhandbook.health.gov.au/resources/tables/table-risk-conditions-and-immunosuppressive-therapies-for-zoster-vaccination-and-eligibility-for-nip-funding

**ATAGI.** COVID-19. Australian Immunisation Handbook, Department of Health, Disability and Ageing (2025a): https://immunisationhandbook.health.gov.au/contents/vaccine-preventable-diseases/covid-19

**ATAGI.** Human papillomavirus (HPV). Australian Immunisation Handbook, Department of Health, Disability and Ageing (2025b): https://immunisationhandbook.health.gov.au/contents/vaccine-preventable-diseases/human-papillomavirus-hpv

**ATAGI.** Pneumococcal disease. Australian Immunisation Handbook, Department of Health, Disability and Ageing (2025c): https://immunisationhandbook.health.gov.au/contents/vaccine-preventable-diseases/pneumococcal-disease

**ATAGI**. Q fever. Australian Immunisation Handbook, Department of Health, Disability and Ageing (2025d): https://immunisationhandbook.health.gov.au/contents/vaccine-preventable-diseases/q-fever

**ATAGI**. Recommendations for vaccination after haematopoietic stem cell transplant in children and adults. Australian Immunisation Handbook, Department of Health, Disability and Ageing (2025e): https://immunisationhandbook.health.gov.au/resources/tables/table-recommendations-for-vaccination-after-haematopoietic-stem-cell-transplant-in-children-and-adults

**ATAGI**. Vaccination for people who are immunocompromised. Australian Immunisation Handbook, Department of Health, Disability and Ageing (2025f): https://immunisationhandbook.health.gov.au/contents/vaccination-for-special-risk-groups/vaccination-for-people-who-are-immunocompromised

**ATAGI**. Zoster (herpes zoster). Australian Immunisation Handbook, Department of Health, Disability and Ageing (2025g): https://immunisationhandbook.health.gov.au/contents/vaccine-preventable-diseases/zoster-herpes-zoster

**Bar-On, Yinon M**., et al. Protection of BNT162b2 vaccine booster against Covid-19 in Israel. New England Journal of Medicine 385.15 (2021): 1393-1400. https://doi.org/10.1056/NEJMoa2114255

**Barrière, J**., et al. Impaired immunogenicity of BNT162b2 anti SARS-CoV-2 vaccine in patients treated for solid tumors. Annals of Oncology 32.8 (2021): 1053-1055. https://doi.org/10.1016/j.annonc.2021.04.019

**Bastidas, Adriana**, et al. Effect of recombinant zoster vaccine on incidence of herpes zoster after autologous stem cell transplantation: a randomized clinical trial. JAMA 322.2 (2019): 123-133. https://doi.org/10.1001/jama.2019.9053

**Bennett, Nancy M**., et al. Use of 13-valent pneumococcal conjugate vaccine and 23-valent pneumococcal polysaccharide vaccine for adults with immunocompromising conditions: recommendations of the Advisory Committee on Immunization Practices. Morbidity and Mortality Weekly Report [MMWR] 61.40 (2012): 816-819.

**Bitterman, Roni**, et al. Influenza vaccines in immunosuppressed adults with cancer. Cochrane Database of Systematic Reviews 2 (2018): CD008983. https://doi.org/10.1002/14651858.CD008983.pub3

**Brisson, M.**, et al. Epidemiology of varicella zoster virus infection in Canada and the United Kingdom. Epidemiology and Infection 127.2 (2001): 305-314. https://doi.org/10.1017/s0950268801005921

**British Lymphology Society (BLS)**. Guidance on Covid-19 and flu vaccinations for people with lymphoedema. BLS and the Lymphoedema Support Network (2023): https://www.thebls.com/documents-library/guidance-on-covid-19-and-flu-vaccinations-for-people-with-lymphoedema

**Cancer Research UK**. Coronavirus (COVID-19). Cancer Research UK (2025): https://www.cancerresearchuk.org/about-cancer/worried-about-cancer/coronavirus-covid-19

**Carpenter, Paul A.**, and Janet A. Englund. How I vaccinate blood and marrow transplant recipients. Blood 127.23 (2016): 2824-2832. https://doi.org/10.1182/blood-2015-12-550475

**Centers for Disease Prevention and Control (CDC)**. Altered immunocompetence. Vaccines & Immunizations, CDC (2024a): https://www.cdc.gov/vaccines/hcp/imz-best-practices/altered-immunocompetence.html

**CDC**. Guillain-Barré syndrome (GBS) and vaccines. Vaccine Safety, CDC (2024b): https://www.cdc.gov/vaccine-safety/about/guillain-barre.html

**CDC**. Pneumococcal vaccine recommendations. Pneumococcal Disease, CDC (2024c): https://www.cdc.gov/pneumococcal/hcp/vaccine-recommendations/index.html

**CDC**. Whooping cough vaccination. Whooping Cough (Pertussis), CDC (2024d): https://www.cdc.gov/pertussis/vaccines/index.html

**CDC**. Immunocompromised travelers. CDC Yellow Book: Health Information for International Travel (2025a): https://www.cdc.gov/yellow-book/hcp/travelers-with-additional-considerations/immunocompromised-travelers.html

**CDC**. Interim clinical considerations for use of COVID-19 vaccines in the United States. COVID-19, CDC (2025b): https://www.cdc.gov/covid/hcp/vaccine-considerations/index.html

**Chong, Curtis R.**, et al. Safety of inactivated influenza vaccine in cancer patients receiving immune checkpoint inhibitors. Clinical Infectious Diseases 70.2 (2020): 193-199. https://doi.org/10.1093/cid/ciz202

**Cordonnier, Catherine**, et al. Vaccination of haemopoietic stem cell transplant recipients: guidelines of the 2017 European Conference on Infections in Leukaemia (ECIL 7). The Lancet Infectious Diseases 19.6 (2019): e200-e212. https://doi.org/10.1016/s1473-3099(18)30600-5

**de la Cámara, R.**, and R. Meisel. Vaccinations. In: Sureda, A., et al. (eds), The EBMT Handbook, Springer (2024): 249-264. https://doi.org/10.1007/978-3-031-44080-9_29

**de Lavallade, Hugues**, et al. Repeated vaccination is required to optimize seroprotection against H1N1 in the immunocompromised host. Haematologica 96.2 (2011): 307-314. https://doi.org/10.3324/haematol.2010.032664

**Department of Health, Disability and Ageing**. NIP childhood and adolescence pneumococcal vaccine provider advice for health professionals. Department of Health, Disability and Ageing (2025): https://www.health.gov.au/resources/publications/nip-childhood-and-adolescence-pneumococcal-vaccine-provider-advice-for-health-professionals

**Dooling, Kathleen L.**, et al. Recommendations of the Advisory Committee on Immunization Practices for use of herpes zoster vaccines. MMWR 67.3 (2018): 103-108. https://doi.org/10.15585/mmwr.mm6703a5

**Douglas, Abby P.**, et al. Ibrutinib may impair serological responses to influenza vaccination. Haematologica 102.10 (2017): e397. https://doi.org/10.3324/haematol.2017.164285

**El-Beyrouty, Claudine**, et al. Pneumococcal vaccination – a literature review and practice guideline update. Pharmacotherapy 42.9 (2022): 724-740. https://doi.org/10.1002/phar.2723

**Eldin, Carole**, et al. From Q fever to *Coxiella burnetii* infection: a paradigm change. Clinical Microbiology Reviews 30.1 (2017): 115-190. https://doi.org/10.1128/cmr.00045-16

**European Centre for Disease Prevention and Control (ECDC)**. COVID-19 vaccination. ECDC (2023): https://www.ecdc.europa.eu/en/covid-19/prevention-and-control/vaccines

**Fry, Sarah E.**, et al. Effectiveness and safety of respiratory syncytial virus vaccine for US adults aged 60 years or older. JAMA Network Open 8.5 (2025): e258322. https://doi.org/10.1001/jamanetworkopen.2025.8322

**Galmiche, Simon**, et al. Immunological and clinical efficacy of COVID-19 vaccines in immunocompromised populations: a systematic review. Clinical Microbiology and Infection 28.2 (2022): 163-177. https://doi.org/10.1016/j.cmi.2021.09.036

**Garassino, M. C.**, et al. The ESMO call to action on COVID-19 vaccinations and patients with cancer: Vaccinate. Monitor. Educate. Annals of Oncology 32.5 (2021): 579-581. https://doi.org/10.1016/j.annonc.2021.01.068

**Garcia Garrido, Hannah M.**, et al. Invasive pneumococcal disease among adults with hematological and solid organ malignancies: a population-based cohort study. International Journal of Infectious Diseases 106 (2021): 237-245. https://doi.org/10.1016/j.ijid.2021.03.072

**Gierke, R.**, et al. Chapter 11: pneumococcal. Manual for the Surveillance of Vaccine-Preventable Diseases, CDC (2025): https://www.cdc.gov/surv-manual/php/table-of-contents/chapter-11-pneumococcal.html

**Grulich, Andrew E.**, et al. Incidence of cancers in people with HIV/AIDS compared with immunosuppressed transplant recipients: a meta-analysis. The Lancet 370.9581 (2007): 59-67. https://doi.org/10.1016/S0140-6736(07)61050-2

**Hall, Victoria**, et al. Protection against SARS-CoV-2 after Covid-19 vaccination and previous infection. New England Journal of Medicine 386.13 (2022): 1207-1220. https://doi.org/10.1056/nejmoa2118691

**Hansson, Erik**, et al. Herpes zoster risk after 21 specific cancers: population-based case-control study. British Journal of Cancer 116.12 (2017): 1643-1651. https://doi.org/10.1038/bjc.2017.124

**Jackson, Lisa A.**, et al. Immunogenicity and safety of a 13-valent pneumococcal conjugate vaccine compared to a 23-valent pneumococcal polysaccharide vaccine in pneumococcal vaccine-naive adults. Vaccine 31.35 (2013): 3577-3584. https://doi.org/10.1016/j.vaccine.2013.04.085

**Joint Committee on Vaccination and Immunisation (JCVI)**. JCVI statement on COVID-19 vaccination in 2025 and spring 2026. Department of Health and Social Care (2024): https://www.gov.uk/government/publications/covid-19-vaccination-in-2025-and-spring-2026-jcvi-advice/

**Joona, Therse Bjorkin**, et al. Influenza vaccination in breast cancer patients during subcutaneous trastuzumab in adjuvant setting. Breast Cancer Research and Treatment 184.1 (2020): 45-52. https://doi.org/10.1007/s10549-020-05815-y

**Kamboj, Mini**, and Monika K. Shah. Vaccination of the stem cell transplant recipient and the hematologic malignancy patient. Infectious Disease Clinics 33.2 (2019): 593-609. https://doi.org/10.1016/j.idc.2019.02.007

**Kamboj, Mini**, et al. Vaccination of adults with cancer: ASCO guideline. Journal of Clinical Oncology 42.14 (2024): 1699-1721. https://doi.org/10.1200/JCO.24.00032

**Karaba, Andrew H.**, et al. Antibody response to respiratory syncytial virus vaccination in immunocompromised persons. JAMA 333.5 (2025): 429-432. https://doi.org/10.1001/jama.2024.25395

**Kearns, Pamela**, et al. Examining the immunological effects of COVID-19 vaccination in patients with conditions potentially leading to diminished immune response capacity – the OCTAVE trial. SSRN (2021). https://doi.org/10.2139/ssrn.3910058

**Kim, Han W.**, et al. Patients with acute myocarditis following mRNA COVID-19 vaccination. JAMA Cardiology 6.10 (2021): 1196-1201. https://doi.org/10.1001/jamacardio.2021.2828

**Kobayashi, Miwako**, DOI. Use of 21-valent pneumococcal conjugate vaccine among US adults: recommendations of the Advisory Committee on Immunization Practices – United States, 2024. MMWR 73.36 (2024): 793-798. https://doi.org/10.15585/mmwr.mm7336a3

**Kuderer, Nicole M.**, et al. Clinical impact of COVID-19 on patients with cancer (CCC19): a cohort study. The Lancet 395.10241 (2020): 1907-1918. https://doi.org/10.1016/s0140-6736(20)31187-9

**Lee, Jason K. H.**, et al. Efficacy and effectiveness of high-dose versus standard-dose influenza vaccination for older adults: a systematic review and meta-analysis. Expert Review of Vaccines 17.5 (2018): 435-443. https://doi.org/10.1080/14760584.2018.1471989.

**Lee, Teresa Sze Mun**, and Karl W. Baumgart. Vaccines and risk of lymphoedema: a case report of a breast cancer patient. Australian Family Physician 41.6 (2012): 404-406.

**Lopez Bernal, Jamie**, et al. Effectiveness of BNT162b2 mRNA vaccine and ChAdOx1 adenovirus vector vaccine on mortality following COVID-19. medRxiv (2021). https://doi.org/10.1101/2021.05.14.21257218

**Lopez-Fauqued, Marta**, et al. Safety profile of the adjuvanted recombinant zoster vaccine in immunocompromised populations: an overview of six trials. Drug Safety 44.7 (2021): 811-823. https://doi.org/10.1007/s40264-021-01076-w

**Mahase, Elisabeth**. Covid-19 booster vaccines: What we know and who's doing what. BMJ 374.8304 (2021): n2082. https://doi.org/10.1136/bmj.n2082

**Marmion, B. P.** Q fever: the long journey to control by vaccination. Medical Journal of Australia, 186.4 (2007): 164-166. https://doi.org/10.5694/j.1326-5377.2007.tb00853.x

**Maurin, M.**, and D. Raoult. Q fever. Clinical Microbiology Reviews 12.4 (1999): 518-553. https://doi.org/10.1128/CMR.12.4.518

**McDonald, Ian**, et al. Comparative systematic review and meta-analysis of reactogenicity, immunogenicity and efficacy of vaccines against SARSCoV-2. NPJ Vaccines 6.1 (2021): 1-14. https://doi.org/10.1038/s41541-021-00336-1

**Meites, E.**, et al. Human papillomavirus vaccination for adults: updated recommendations of the Advisory Committee on Immunization Practices. MMWR 68.32 (2019): 698-702. https://doi.org/10.15585/mmwr.mm6832a3

**Miller, P. D. E.**, et al. Joint consensus statement on the vaccination of adult and paediatric haematopoietic stem cell transplant recipients: prepared on behalf of the British Society of Blood and Marrow Transplantation and Cellular Therapy (BSBMTCT), the Children's Cancer and Leukaemia Group (CCLG), and British Infection Association (BIA). Journal of Infection 86.1 (2023): 1-8. https://doi.org/10.1016/j.jinf.2022.11.005

**Montgomery, Jay**, et al. Myocarditis following immunization with mRNA COVID-19 vaccines in members of the US military. JAMA Cardiology 6.10 (2021): 1202-1206. https://doi.org/10.1001/jamacardio.2021.2833

**Munro, Clara**. Covid-19: 40% of patients with weakened immune system mount lower response to vaccines. BMJ 374 (2021): n2098. https://doi.org/10.1136/bmj.n2098

**National Comprehensive Cancer Network (NCCN)**. NCCN guidelines for the prevention and treatment of cancer-related infections, version 1.2025. NCCN (2025): https://www.nccn.org/guidelines/guidelines-detail?category=3&id=1457

**Pollyea, Daniel A.**, et al. Utility of influenza vaccination for oncology patients. Journal of Clinical Oncology 28.14 (2010): 2481-2490. https://doi.org/10.1200/jco.2009.26.6908

**Public Health Agency of Canada**. Immunization of immunocompromised persons. Canadian Immunization Guide, PHAC (2024): https://www.canada.ca/en/public-health/services/publications/healthy-living/canadian-immunization-guide-part-3-vaccination-specific-populations/page-8-immunization-immunocompromised-persons.html

**Ram, Ron**, et al. Safety and immunogenicity of the BNT162b2 mRNA Covid-19 vaccine in patients after allogeneic HCT or CD19-based CART therapy – a single center prospective cohort study. Transplantation and Cellular Therapy 27.9 (2021): 788-794. https://doi.org/10.1016/j.jtct.2021.06.024

**Raoult, D.**, et al. Acute and chronic Q fever in patients with cancer. Clinical Infectious Diseases 14.1 (1992): 127-130. https://doi.org/10.1093/clinids/14.1.127

**Riedel, Andreas**, et al. Immunological consequences of CAR T-cell therapy: an analysis of infectious complications and immune reconstitution. Blood Advances 9.13 (2025): 3149-3158. https://doi.org/10.1182/bloodadvances.2024015346

**Roberts, Matthew B.**, et al. Clinical effectiveness of conjugate pneumococcal vaccination in hematopoietic stem cell transplantation recipients. Biology of Blood and Marrow Transplantation 26.2 (2020): 421-427. https://doi.org/10.1016/j.bbmt.2019.10.006

**Robilotti, Elizabeth**, et al. Epidemiology of *Bordetella pertussis* among patients with cancer. Clinical Infectious Diseases 70.10 (2020): 2237-2238. https://doi.org/10.1093/cid/ciz815

**Rubin, Lorry G.**, et al. 2013 IDSA clinical practice guideline for vaccination of the immunocompromised host. Clinical Infectious Diseases 58.3 (2014): e44-e100. https://doi.org/10.1093/cid/cit684

**Sampathkumar, Priya**, et al. Herpes zoster (shingles) and postherpetic neuralgia. Mayo Clinic Proceedings 84.3 (2009): 274-280. https://doi.org/10.4065/84.3.274

**Sander, Robert**. Otitis externa: a practical guide to treatment and prevention. American Family Physician 63.5 (2001): 927-936.

**Seth, T.**, et al. Preventing pneumococcal infections in patients with hematological malignancies: a review of evidence and recommendations based on modified Delphi consensus. Frontiers in Oncology 15 (2025): 1-15. https://doi.org/10.3389/fonc.2025.1546641

**Shapiro, R. A.**, et al. A randomized, controlled, double-blind, cross-over, clinical trial of Q fever vaccine in selected Queensland abattoirs. Epidemiology & Infection 104.2 (1990): 267-273. https://doi.org/10.1017/s0950268800059446

**Shay, David K.**, et al. Myocarditis occurring after immunization with mRNA-based COVID-19 vaccines. JAMA Cardiology 6.10 (2021): 1115-1117. https://doi.org/10.1001/jamacardio.2021.2821

**Shigayeva, Altynay**, et al. Invasive pneumococcal disease among immunocompromised persons: implications for vaccination programs. Clinical Infectious Diseases 62.2 (2016): 139-147. https://doi.org/10.1093/cid/civ803

**Standish, L. J.**, et al. Immune defects in breast cancer patients after radiotherapy. Journal of the Society for Integrative Oncology 6.3 (2008): 110-121. https://doi.org/10.2310/7200.2008.0018

**Sun, Clare**, et al. Seasonal influenza vaccination in patients with chronic lymphocytic leukemia treated with ibrutinib. JAMA Oncology 2.12 (2016): 1656-1657. https://doi.org/10.1001/jamaoncol.2016.2437

**Therapeutic Goods Administration (TGA)**. Australian product information – Q-VAX® Q fever vaccine and Q-VAX® skin test (version 7). Department of Health, Disability and Ageing (2019), available at https://www.tga.gov.au/resources/artg/100517

**UK Health Security Agency (UKHSA)**. Immunisation against infectious disease. The Green Book, UKHSA (2025): https://www.gov.uk/government/collections/immunisation-against-infectious-disease-the-green-book

**Vijenthira, Abi**, et al. Outcomes of patients with hematologic malignancies and COVID-19: a systematic review and meta-analysis of 3377 patients. Blood 136.25 (2020): 2881-2892. https://doi.org/10.1182/blood.2020008824

**van Deursen, Anna M. M.**, et al. Immunogenicity of the 13-valent pneumococcal conjugate vaccine in older adults with and without comorbidities in the community-acquired pneumonia immunization trial in adults (CAPiTA). Clinical Infectious Diseases 65.5 (2017): 787-795. https://doi.org/10.1093/cid/cix419

**Vink, Peter**, et al. Immunogenicity and safety of the adjuvanted recombinant zoster vaccine in patients with solid tumors, vaccinated before or during chemotherapy: a randomized trial. Cancer 125.8 (2019): 1301-1312. https://doi.org/10.1002/cncr.31909

**Voysey, Merryn**, et al. Safety and efficacy of the ChAdOx1 nCoV-19 vaccine (AZD1222) against SARS-CoV-2: an interim analysis of four randomised controlled trials in Brazil, South Africa, and the UK. The Lancet 397.10269 (2021a): 99-111. https://doi.org/10.1016/S0140-6736(20)32661-1

**Voysey, Merryn**, et al. Single-dose administration and the influence of the timing of the booster dose on immunogenicity and efficacy of ChAdOx1 nCoV-19 (AZD1222) vaccine: a pooled analysis of four randomised trials. The Lancet 397.10277 (2021b): 881-891. https://doi.org/10.1016/S0140-6736(21)00432-3

**Waissengrin, Barliz**, et al. Short-term safety of the BNT162b2 mRNA COVID-19 vaccine in patients with cancer treated with immune checkpoint inhibitors. The Lancet Oncology 22.5 (2021): 581-583. https://doi.org/10.1016/s1470-2045(21)00155-8

**Wersal, Cornelia**, et al. Long-term changes in blood counts after intraoperative radiotherapy for breast cancer—single center experience and review of the literature. Translational Cancer Research 8.5 (2019): 1882-1903. https://doi.org/10.21037/tcr.2019.09.05

**Yu, Xiaocong**, et al. Neutralizing antibodies derived from the B cells of 1918 influenza pandemic survivors. Nature 455.7212 (2008): 532-536. https://doi.org/10.1038/nature07231

**Zent, Clive S.**, et al. Short term results of vaccination with adjuvanted recombinant varicella zoster glycoprotein E during initial BTK inhibitor therapy for CLL or lymphoplasmacytic lymphoma. Leukemia 35.6 (2021): 1788-1791. https://doi.org/10.1038/s41375-020-01074-4

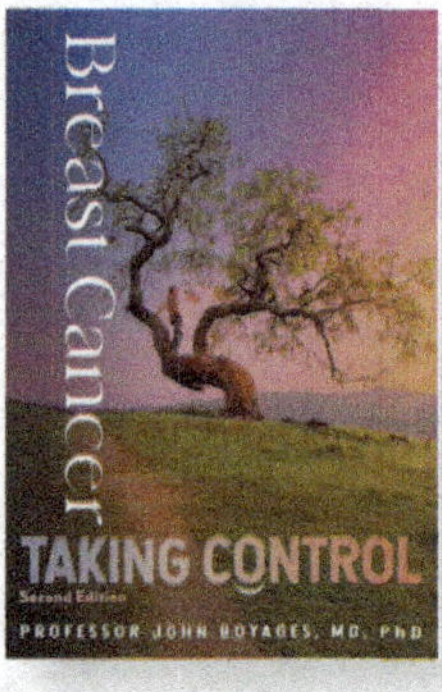
Breast Cancer
TAKING CONTROL
Second Edition
PROFESSOR JOHN BOYAGES, MD, PhD

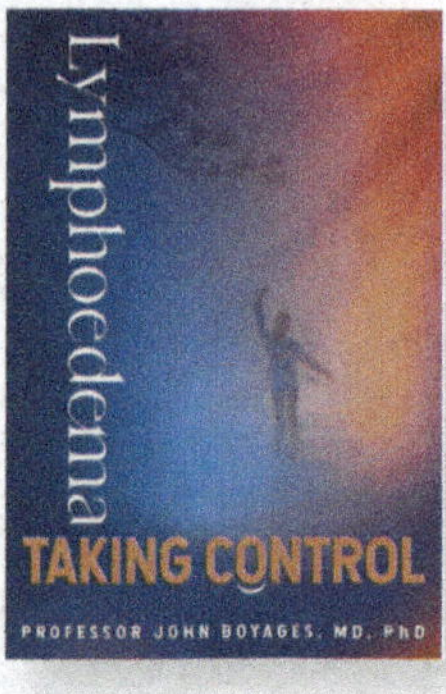
Lymphoedema
TAKING CONTROL
PROFESSOR JOHN BOYAGES, MD, PhD

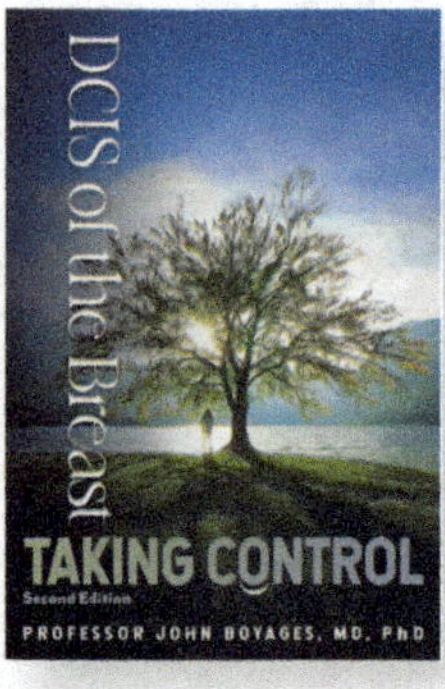
DCIS of the Breast
TAKING CONTROL
Second Edition
PROFESSOR JOHN BOYAGES, MD, PhD

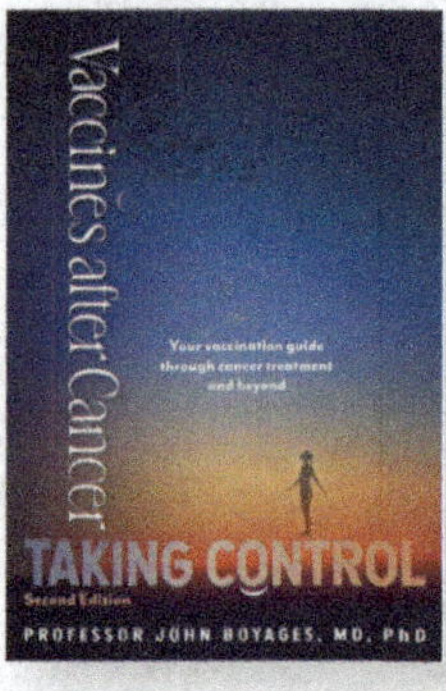
Vaccines after Cancer
Your vaccination guide through cancer treatment and beyond
TAKING CONTROL
Second Edition
PROFESSOR JOHN BOYAGES, MD, PhD

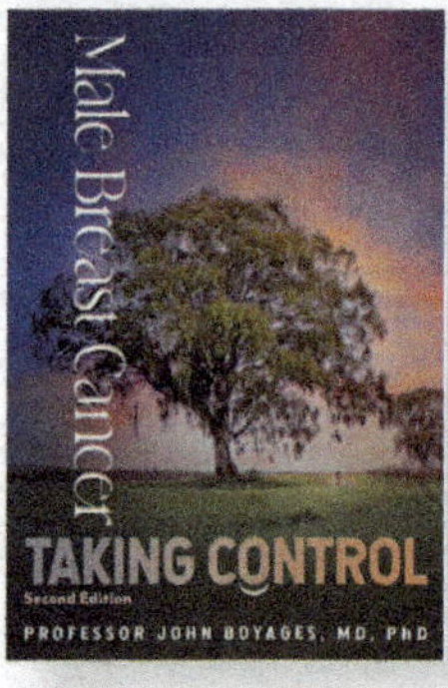
Male Breast Cancer
TAKING CONTROL
Second Edition
PROFESSOR JOHN BOYAGES, MD, PhD

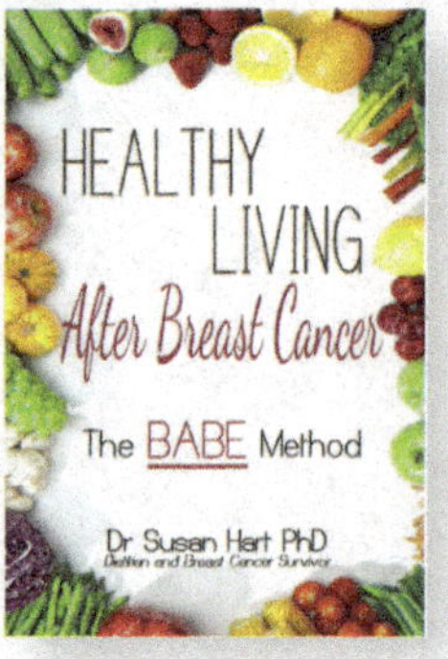
HEALTHY
LIVING
After Breast Cancer
The BABE Method
Dr Susan Hart PhD